Interpersonal Interaction in Nursing

Basic Concepts in Nurse-Patient Communication

Virgil Parsons, R.N.
San Jose State University

Nancy Sanford, R.N., M.S.
Independent Practitioner in Nursing Education

Addison-Wesley Publishing Company
Medical/Nursing Division
Menlo Park, California • Reading, Massachusetts
London • Amsterdam • Don Mills, Ontario • Sydney

The Addison-Wesley p.r.n. Module Series in Nursing Concepts and Skills

Margaret W. Rochin, R.N.
San Jose State University
Martha A. Thompson, R.N.
San Jose State University
Consulting Editors

Photographs by Lea Meyer

Grateful acknowledgment is given to the following publishers and authors for permission to quote materials from their books: Lawrence M. Brammer, *The Helping Relationship: Process and Skills,* © 1973. pp. 81–87. Adapted by permission of Prentice-Hall, Inc., Englewood Cliffs, New Jersey. / Carolyn E. Carlson, Ed. "Trust in the Nurse-Patient Relationship," *Behavioral Concepts and Nursing Interventions,* © 1970. Philadelphia: J. B. Lippincott Company. / Maxie D. Dunnam, "Cycles in My Life," in *Dancing at My Funeral,* 1973, reprinted by permission of the author. / Gerard Egan. *Encounter: Group Processes for Interpersonal Growth,* © 1970. Belmont, California: Brooks/Cole Publishing Co. / Gerard Egan, Ed. "One Small-Group Leader's Paradoxical Problems of Becoming a Member of His Own Group," *Encounter Groups: Basic Readings,* © 1971, Belmont, California: Brooks/Cole Publishing Co. / T. S. Eliot, from "Little Gidding" in *Four Quartets* by T. S. Eliot, copyright, 1943, by T. S. Eliot; copyright, 1971, by Esme Valerie Eliot. Reprinted by permission of Harcourt Brace Jovanovich, Inc. / David W. Johnson, *Reaching Out: Interpersonal Effectiveness and Self-actualization,* © 1972. Reprinted by permission of Prentice-Hall, Inc., Englewood Cliffs, New Jersey. / L. L. Langley, Ira R. Telford, and John B. Cristensen, *Dynamic Anatomy and Physiology,* Fourth Edition, © 1974. "Light Reflexes," Figure 12–17, p. 321. New York City: McGraw-Hill Book Company. / Garland K. Lewis, *Nurse-Patient Communication,* 2nd Edition, 1973, Wm. C. Brown Company Publishers, Dubuque, Iowa. / Joseph Luft. *Of Human Interaction,* © 1969. Palo Alto, California: National Press Books. / Maureen J. O'Brien: *Communications and Relationships in Nursing,* ed. 2, St. Louis, 1974, The C. V. Mosby Co. / Ronal G. Poland: *Human Experience: A Psychology of Growth,* St. Louis, 1974, The C. V. Mosby Co. / V. Satir. *Peoplemaking.* Palo Alto, California: Science and Behavior Books, 1972. / *Webster's New World Dictionary, Popular Library Paperback Edition.* Copyright © 1975 by William Collins + World Publishing Co., Inc.

Library of Congress Catalog Card No. 77-87342.

ISBN 0-201-05551-1
BCDEFGHIJ-AL-79

Addison-Wesley Publishing Company
Medical/Nursing Division
2725 Sand Hill Road
Menlo Park, California 94025

Personal Resources in Nursing Module Series

Series Foreword

The p.r.n. Series grew out of our desire to improve the quality of instruction in nursing and to make learning more individualized and productive. Self-contained, independent learning units (modules) provide an alternative educational method which helps to achieve these goals as well as provide broader learning experiences for a greater number of students. The editors have also found that this teaching approach increases flexibility in the instructional process and personal interaction between student and teacher.

The topics for the series were selected because they represent major concepts which are basic to nursing education regardless of curriculum level or structure. The series consists of a number of independent learning units, each dealing with a single concept or topic. Each module is self-contained. Required learning is reflected in behaviorally stated goals and objectives. Content is based on a synthesis of material from various resources, and mastery of content is measured by entry and exit evaluation tools. Instructional activities are designed to actively involve the learner. Based on these criteria, the editors believe that the modules of the p.r.n. Series will facilitate the teaching/learning process for both student and teacher.

Margaret W. Rochin
Martha A. Thompson

Preface

Anne Morrow Lindbergh has stated that "good communication is as stimulating as black coffee, and just as hard to sleep after." An essential component of providing nursing care is being able to communicate skillfully with the client in a variety of settings. It is also necessary that the nurse have enough self-awareness and understanding of others to know when the communication should be stimulating and when it should help the client in feeling quiet and at peace.

Our goal for this book is to assist nursing students and practitioners in the development of increased self-awareness and skill in effective communication. It has been written in such a way as to consistently involve the reader in the process of gaining new knowledge about self, and the use of self in communication. Each unit includes objectives, a pretest, and a posttest for self-measuring the learning achieved. The reader is led through experiences in the theory of awareness and communication, and then given direction in how to apply that knowledge through nursing interventions. The concepts are basic, and they are crucial to successful nursing.

The topics are organized (ordered) with the intent of creating a flow in the reader's learning. An overall focus is self-awareness, for which the stage is set by looking at *Self-Disclosure* in the nursing process. *Thoughts and Feelings* are explored next, with an emphasis on differentiation of these two concepts. Based on these first two units, *Trust* is presented as a foundation for the nurse-client relationship; this is followed by *Listening,* which reinforces trust as a basis for nurse and client working together. *Body Language, Support,* and *Feedback* are then discussed as three interrelated components of therapeutic communication. Lastly, *Termination* pinpoints the need for dealing with separation anxiety and for appropriately ending the nurse-client relationship when the "work" is done.

These units can be used by the beginning nursing student in the order presented. They can also be read and used individually and independently, according to need. For example, the nurse involved in caring for women in childbirth may benefit by reading the unit on *Support* first. A nursing student studying community health practice might wish to read the unit on *Trust* before making a home visit. If, while caring for a client, some barriers seem to exist, it might be helpful to read the *Listening* and *Feedback* units. It is intended that nursing faculty will use the book as an aid to clinical experience, asking students to read various units according to foci and problems that develop in the process of planning and giving nursing care.

We extend appreciation to our students and colleagues at San Jose State University, Department of Nursing. Special thanks to Fay Bower and Margaret Rochin for their encouragement and support in the development of these lessons. Gratitude is due Mary M. Murphy for editing assistance.

Virgil Parsons
Nancy Sanford

Contents

Thoughts and Feelings

DIRECTIONS

1. Complete the pretest. If you answer all the questions correctly, you may choose to complete the unit on thoughts and feelings for added enrichment and knowledge.

2. After the pretest, complete the activities as directed. The activities and exercises should be completed in the order presented.

3. In order to complete the unit, you will need a pencil or pen. No other materials are needed.

4. A posttest will be given at the end of the unit. Successful completion of this test is necessary for you to have met the unit objectives.

OBJECTIVES Upon completion of this unit on thoughts and feelings, the learner will be able to:

1. Define thoughts.
2. Describe the process of thought (mental activity).
3. Identify three activities related to thought.
4. Define feelings.
5. Describe three kinds of feelings.
6. Identify at least five physiological effects of feelings.
7. Describe four ways in which feelings are handled.
8. Differentiate thoughts and feelings.
9. Explain the relatedness of thoughts, feelings, and behavior.
10. Describe one's own thoughts and feelings in response to a given situation.

Pretest

True (T) or False (F)

_____ 1. Thoughts refer to those activities carried on by the brain, otherwise known as "mental activity."

_____ 2. Thinking implies reasoning, experiencing sensations, and use of ideas.

_____ 3. Thinking is a potential for growth and development that is present at birth.

_____ 4. Cognitive behavior is always logical, although not directly observable.

_____ 5. The "mind's eye" refers to the development of attitudes and ways of interpreting the world.

_____ 6. The "higher mental processes" are devoted to discrimination and learning.

_____ 7. Fixed ideas assist a person in creative problem-solving.

_____ 8. Feelings refer to an idea or awareness of an emotion.

_____ 9. Feelings include the ability to experience physical sensation.

_____ 10. Feelings tend to be very difficult to identify and express.

____ 11. Affective behavior is synonymous with feeling.

____ 12. A feeling labeled as pleasant is said to have "affective tone."

____ 13. A person who suppresses feelings is inhibited in functioning, but is usually quite content.

____ 14. Being aware of a patient's sensations would assist you in planning nursing care.

____ 15. Feelings can be need states manifested as tension.

____ 16. Bodily processes are little affected by the experience of feelings and emotions.

____ 17. Expressing feelings obliquely occurs when an individual negates responsibility for an emotion or sensation.

____ 18. Denial and internalization of feelings can cause physical symptoms and problems.

____ 19. Acting out feelings implies transfer of expression to a more appropriate person or object.

____ 20. It is always best to take responsibility for feelings and express them directly.

Pretest Answers

1. True	2. False	3. True	4. False	5. False	6. True
7. False	8. False	9. True	10. True	11. True	12. False
13. False	14. True	15. True	16. False	17. True	
18. True	19. False	20. False			

INTRODUCTION

Thoughts and feelings, and the difference between them, may not seem important to study. However, people often confuse the two. Have you not often heard a person say, "I feel . . .," when he or she is about to state an opinion or idea? It is socially acceptable to use this manner of expression, but it does not make communication very clear. For example, if a person says, "I feel that abortion should not be legal." is the person indicating that:

1. his or her emotions or sensations are such that he or she cannot tolerate the "taking of a human life,"

or,

2. his or her exploration of the problem of unwanted pregnancy has led the person to believe that abortion is not an appropriate solution?

Another illustration of the difficulty in knowing the difference between thoughts and feelings is with students just beginning to study communication and interpersonal relations. When asked to describe a feeling, they often state a thought. For example, instead of saying, "I felt angry and humiliated," the individual might say, "I don't think you should have been so abrupt with me. I feel you were very rude!"

By the end of this module, you should have an understanding of thoughts and feelings, and the importance of differentiating the two. This knowledge will increase your self-awareness and assist you in establishing and maintaining effective interpersonal relationships.

THOUGHTS

Thoughts are but dreams till
their effects be tried. *SHAKESPEARE*

First, let us consider thoughts—those activities carried on by the brain, otherwise known as "mental activity." Take a few minutes and consider the word *thought*. Write several words that readily come to mind. Blanks are provided on the next page.

1.	6.
2.	7.
3.	8.
4.	9.
5.	10.

Possible responses are:

thinking	brain	know
reason	mental	knowledge
rational	image	logic
idea	believe	logical
concept	belief	sensible
cognitive	opinion	rationale
mind	notion	
meditate	understand	

Did your list include others? Based on what you wrote and the words listed, formulate a brief definition for *thought.*

Thought is:

Compare your definition with that from a dictionary:

1. the act or process of thinking
2. the power of reasoning
3. idea, concept, and so on
4. attention; consideration *(Webster's New World Dictionary, Popular Library Paperback Edition.* Copyright © 1975 by Williams Collins + World Publishing Co. Inc.).

Key words that should stand out are:

thinking – reasoning – idea – concept

Man is a thinking being,
whether he will or no:
all he can do is to turn
his thoughts the best way. *SIR W. TEMPLE*

Thoughts, then, are the direct results of thinking, using the mind to reason. According to Poland, thinking is one of the potentials for growth and development that is present in humans at birth (Poland, 1974, p. 16).

> Thinking: This at-birth potential is often referred to as *cognitive behavior*. Cognition, as in the words *recognize* and *recognition*, has to do with intellect, the "use of the mind," whether it is logical or illogical. Thinking is not directly observable, although an individual human may experience within himself what is called thinking (Poland, 1974, p. 13).

The potential for thinking is inherited, but whether and how it is actualized depends on the interaction between the potential and many environmental factors. For example, effective thinking (mental activity) develops through learning and appropriate stimulation to solve problems.

It is the mind that maketh good or ill,
That maketh wretch or happy, rich or poor. *SPENSER*

Thinking goes on continually in the brain. Part of mental activity is the internal pictures that pass through the "mind's eye." These may be fantasies, images from the past, or representations of needs and wants. Many needs are represented mentally before they are expressed in behavioral terms. For example, you might picture candy, then experience the sensation labeled hunger, and then ingest the "goodies" previously pictured in the mind. The reverse (hunger–"picture" food– eating) is also possible. By paying attention to these inner pictures, you can get a better sense of your needs and desires, and exert control over your behavior, making it more congruent with what is going on inside of you.

"Mind's Eye" Exercise To illustrate the "mind's eye," let your mind focus on your favorite food–a thick, juicy hamburger; fried chicken; chocolate cake; whatever. Imagine just how this food looks in its ready-to-eat form, just waiting for you to pounce on it and devour it. Now, check out what sensations you are experiencing. Unless you have just eaten and are thoroughly satiated, you should be feeling a little hungry. Are you? (You may want to stop working for a minute and eat a little something so that the aroused hunger does not interfere with your continued concentration on this module.)

Another form of mental activity occurs in the process of growing up, when people develop habits of thought, ideas and attitudes, and ways of interpreting the world. These ideas and habits of thought are introjected from parents and the child's world, and they provide a basis for the person's philosophy of living. Often the attitudes become fixed and are not reevaluated as the child enters the adult world; and since they are integrated into the personality and influence behavior in later life, individuals may not be aware how they color their experience, limit their alternatives, or restrict their modes of experiencing life. Becoming conscious of these thought patterns, and accepting only those that fit your being of the present, is a most important way to increase your self-awareness and enable you to live and experience the "here and now" world.

Take a few minutes to examine some of your own ideas and attitudes about premarital sex and answer the following questions.

1. An *idea or attitude* that I have is:

2. This influences my life now by:

3. A *fixed* idea or attitude I have is:

4. This fixed thought influences my life now by:

There are no "right" answers. The goal is to be more aware of your ideas, attitudes, images from the past, and so on, and to look at how these influence your current functioning and life-style.

Thoughts and thinking are also related to another very important activity—learning. Experts concerned with learning theory place emphasis on one's ability to perform complex cognitive processes—thinking, language use, and problem-solving. The outer core of the brain, the cerebral cortex, controls discrimination, choice, learning, and thinking—the "higher mental processes." Thinking, as a cognitive form of behavior, is characterized by the use of concepts, which are *symbolic* thoughts that stand for a class of objects, events, or ideas with common properties. Because thought is symbolic, it can range widely in its content. Language is a major source of symbols and concepts used in thinking; thus, language and thought are closely related.

Some concepts are symbols for concrete objects, such as *chair*; and some, like *language*, convey abstract meaning. Put the concepts listed below into two groups—concrete and abstract.

pain	health	pill
dog	justice	button
syringe	God	nursing
	nurse	

Concrete	**Abstract**
1.	1.
2.	2.
3.	3.
4.	4.
5.	5.

ANSWERS

Concrete	**Abstract**
1. dog	1. pain
2. syringe	2. health
3. nurse	3. justice
4. pill	4. God
5. button	5. nursing

Now try out your ability at problem-solving and creative thinking. First, fill in the blanks for normal and novel use of a common object.

Tool	Normal Use	Novel Use
1. box	as a container	
2. hammer	to drive nails	
3. knife		to pry open a lid

POSSIBLE ANSWERS

1. as a table
2. as a weapon
3. to cut or slice

Next, without exchanging the glasses, how can you arrange the pattern so that empty and full glasses alternate, that is, empty-full-empty, and so on?

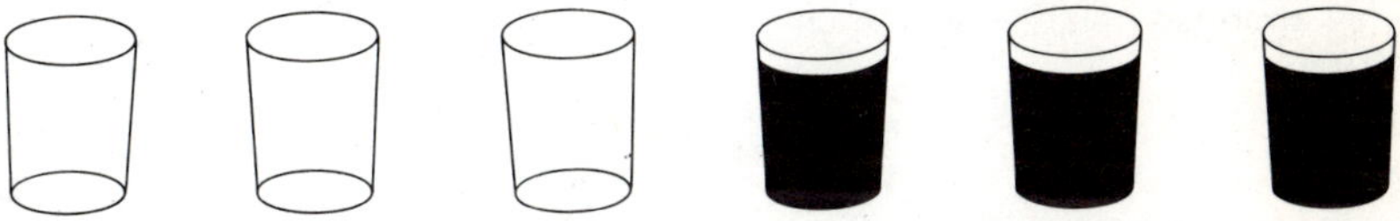

ANSWER

Lift the middle full glass, pour it into the middle empty one, and replace the now empty glass between the full ones.

FEELINGS

Passions, like seas, will have
their ebbs and flows. *LEE*

Now we will explore feelings. As you did for thoughts, think of the word, *feeling*, and list words that occur to you.

1.	6.
2.	7.
3.	8.
4.	9.
5.	10.

Possible responses:

feel	sensitivity	tension	moving
sensation	perception	excitement	desire
emotion	sympathy	fear	affect
touch	anger	hate	
sense	thrill	love	
awareness	sentiment	stress	

Did you think of others? Write a definition for *feeling.*

Feeling is:

Now consider the following dictionary definition:

1. the sense of touch
2. the ability to experience physical sensation
3. an awareness; sensation
4. an emotion
5. (plural) sensitivities (for example, hurt *feelings*)
6. sympathy; pity *(Webster's New World Dictionary, Popular Library Paperback Edition.* Copyright © 1975 by William Collins + World Publishing Co., Inc.).

Words to keep in mind are:

sense of touch—physical sensation—emotion—sensitivities

Of all the tyrants the world affords,
Our own affections are the fiercest lords. *EARL OF STERLING*

Feelings include emotions (such as anger, sadness, love), sensations (such as pain, pressure, cold) and the tensions of need states (such as hunger, sexual excitement, fatigue). Life without feelings would be dull and colorless; yet they are very difficult to identify, understand, express, and utilize constructively.

Like *thinking*, Poland considers *feeling* and *perceiving* to be preconditions of behavior development that are typically present at birth (Poland, 1974, p. 16).

> Feeling: This genetically based potential is sometimes called *affective behavior*, and it has to do with a wide variety of behavior ranging from sadness and depression through happiness and ecstatic joy. Feelings are not directly observable, although they often may be expressed through action (Poland, 1974, p. 13). *and*
>
> Perceiving: The equipment of perception is a part of all we inherit from our biological parents. Most of us inherit ears and eyes that work, tongues that are able to taste, noses that can sniff and smell a great variety of aromas, and nerve endings in the skin that help us to know when we touch or are touched. Perceiving is an intricate behavior that has a clear biological base, the base of sensing. We must sense sounds, odors, pressures, tastes, warmth and coolth before they can be perceived (Poland, 1974, p. 13).

Both of these descriptions pertain to your study of the three kinds of feelings discussed here—emotions, sensations, tensions of need states.

Emotions can be described as pleasurable states, such as warmth or love, and unpleasant states, such as anger or sadness. When we label a feeling as pleasant or not, we are referring to the *affective tone*. Affect is the range of emotion we feel and experience, and many emotional terms express the intensity (amount of affect) of the experience. For example, the differences in intensity are noted by words such as anger-rage, fear-terror, pain-agony, and so on. Emotions are natural and vital to our psychological well-being, and learning to express them can be a great source of joy. The person who suppresses feelings is inhibited in functioning, and often suffers "mental illness" (depression) or physical problems (ulcer).

Identify the emotions associated with the thoughts by filling in the blanks with an appropriate feeling. There are no absolutely right answers—just those that "fit" with the thoughts and are correct for you.

1. I looked forward to nursing for years. Now I'm finally in the program and we aren't doing enough nursing. Just studying books and theory. I feel ________________ .

2. There I was sitting in the student union trying to look "cool" and I spilled my coke all over me and the table. Man, I felt really ________________ .

3. I didn't do too well on the last test, but my other classes seem to be going okay. I'm not too sure. I feel ________________ about school.

POSSIBLE ANSWERS

1. frustrated-angry

2. embarrassed-humiliated

3. anxious-upset

Feelings include sensations; most directly related to our discussion are the sense impressions of pressure, pain, and temperature (cold-hot). Experiencing these sensations allows you to perceive, and provides important clues, to your functioning and state of being. Pressure can warn you to move an extremity before circulation is impeded severely, pain lets you know that all is not right with a vital organ or part of the body, and intense warmth suggests the presence of infection. Being aware of, and attending to, these feelings will help you correct malfunctionings in the body before they become irreversible.

Briefly describe an example of how being aware of a client's sensation would assist you in planning care for this person.

1. Pressure:

2. Pain:

3. Temperature:

POSSIBLE ANSWERS—these are only a few

1. Periodically changing the position of an immobilized patient to prevent stress ulcers (bedsores). Making sure casts do not inhibit circulation and blood flow.

2. Knowing how much or how little pain-relief medication to give (assuming the physician's order indicates a range of dose). Assessing a client's condition or extent of injury.

3. Assessing need for encouraging fluids. Keeping the client's room at a temperature conducive to comfort and appropriate warmth.

Also, feelings can be need states manifested as tension. These too are major indications of functioning or warning to take measures to maintain high-level wellness. Hunger, fatigue, sexual excitement, and so on, all give rise to behavior that protects you from deprivation and maladaptation.

Write the behavior that should follow the tension of the listed need states.

1. Hunger:

2. Fatigue:

3. Sexual arousal:

The first two answers were likely obvious; the third, not so easy to answer. This illustrates that not all need states are simply or easily attended to, even if awareness exists.

> The human heart is often the victim of the sensations of the moment; success intoxicates it to presumption, and disappointment dejects and terrifies it. *VOLNEY*

Very often, feelings and emotions are manifested by symptoms you experience in bodily processes. One of these, already mentioned, is muscle tension. There are also changes in blood pressure and in the distribution of blood between body surface and interior, for example, blushing with embarrassment or getting "hot under the collar." The heart rate alters with the experience of excitement or fear. Feelings can be detected by a test, the galvanic skin response, which measures electrical changes that take place on the skin. This test is a sensitive indicator of changes in emotional or feeling states. Feelings also bring about alterations in respiration, perspiration, pupils, and gastrointestinal motility.

List at least five physiological effects of feelings and emotions.

1.

2.

3.

4.

5.

If you had difficulty completing this exercise, review the preceding paragraph to find your answers.

All our actions take
Their hues from the complexion of the heart,
As landscapes their variety from light. *W. T. BACON*

Feelings are expressed in some form of behavior—verbal and/or nonverbal. The way we express feelings and emotions is perhaps the most frequent source of problems in interpersonal relationships. These problems arise not because we have the feelings, but because we have difficulty experiencing or expressing them fully, with affect, or constructively.

To deal with a feeling, one must first accept responsibility for experiencing it. When a person tries to negate this responsibility, the expression of feelings most often occurs in *oblique (indirect)* ways. If, for instance, your roommate comes bopping home wearing an article of clothing "borrowed" from you when you were out to class, you might be irritated. Obliquely, you could handle this feeling in one of the following ways:

1. Projecting feeling on another: "You seem upset."
2. Questioning another: "Didn't you realize that belongs to me?"
3. Accusing another: "You care only about what you want!"
4. Sarcasm: "Hell will freeze over before you change your ways."
5. Name-calling: "You inconsiderate jerk!"

6. Invalidating another: "I guess you're too immature to know you should have asked first."

7. Approval-disapproval expressions: "You're terrific" or "You're stupid."

Thus, only if you take responsibility for the feeling will you be able to express it clearly. Taking responsibility is being accountable; and since feelings guide actions and behavior, then each of us must accept responsibility for our own feelings.

Another way feelings are handled is through *denial* and/or *internalization*. People do this because it seems easier than acknowledging and dealing with their feelings. Using this method, a person does not admit to self or others that the feeling even exists. The result is that the feeling is internalized (suppressed or repressed), and very likely wreaks havoc on the individual's body (ulcers, colitis, and so on). This is true most often for negative feelings such as anger or sadness. Your irritation with your roommate regarding the borrowed clothing could be denied and held in—"No, I'm not at all upset that you wore my shirt and ripped it up the back."—and could be expressed through a severe headache or "knot" in the stomach. Do you recognize that you ever do this?

Acting out refers to another method of "nondealing" with feelings. This is usually done in the form of *displacement*, whereby a feeling is transferred to a more acceptable-to-self (or available) substitute person or object. If this mechanism occurred with the roommate/clothing situation, you would direct the feeling at something or someone else. You might slam the door or break a dish; you might tell-off a friend (and won't that person be surprised) or kick a dog. Displacement can often set up a chain-reaction series of events, which can be cyclical, for example, your teacher yells at you, you take it out on a patient, the patient yells at a nurse aide, the aide takes it out on a coworker, the coworker yells at the head nurse, the head nurse takes it out on a doctor, the doctor yells at the supervisor, the supervisor takes it out on your teacher, and your teacher asks, confused, "Why me?" Acting out is also evident in some antisocial or criminal behavior where the individual is frustrated or "mad at the world" and expresses it through vandalism or destructive acts.

A fourth, and the most healthy, way to handle feelings is by *taking responsibility and fully experiencing them.* This means that the individual will go through a process (sometimes very quickly) of:

1. *Identifying the feeling.* This requires recognizing and acknowledging the emotion, sensation or tension. For example, returning to the borrowed article of clothing, you might say to yourself, "My shirt is gone; J. likely borrowed it. I feel unsettled and a little anxious."

2. *Labeling and describing.* In this step, you need to correctly differentiate which of many possible feelings you are experiencing, for example, "What I am feeling right now is irritation and anger. Grrrr!"

3. *Expressing and externalizing.* This act can be either verbal or nonverbal. Verbally, you might express the feeling by a specific label, for example, "I feel angry"; or use other words or figures of speech to describe the feeling, for example, "I feel like my blood's boiling" or "I am really bugged." The clearest way is to label the feeling specifically.

Nonverbal behavior might be physical activity that is congruent with, or supports, the verbal expression, for example, clenching of fists and grimacing; or it might occur by itself without verbal behavior, for example, wailing and jumping up and down. Usually, it is most effective to use words along with or to follow up nonverbal expression.

4. *Accepting responsibility and expression.* This part of the process requires that the person "own" the feeling and do "working through" as directly as possible. When your roommate came home, you might state, "J., I need to tell you something. I feel angry that you borrowed my shirt without asking. I had planned to wear it and it wasn't here." It is best to stop with a brief statement and allow J. to respond. You might be surprisingly informed, "I didn't wear your shirt. It's in the dirty clothes where you put it." If you allow for this possibility, you will save yourself much embarrassment (another unpleasant feeling).

Allowing J. to respond also might result in "I'm sorry. I can understand your irritation. I won't do it again." Unless this is the forty-fourth time you have heard this, it would likely be best to accept the apology and let the matter drop. A definite benefit of the direct expression is that you have clarified the relationship and agreement with J. J. now knows that it is not okay with you to borrow your clothing without asking permission. Most important, you have fully experienced your feeling of anger and can let it go without it interfering with the continued relationship.

It needs to be pointed out that there will be times when it would be inappropriate, impossible, or unsafe to directly express a feeling. These include situations when:

1. You assess that the other person will be unable or unwilling to accept your expression or be deeply hurt by it. If J. came home obviously depressed about having failed a test, it would be very heartless of you to give vent to your feelings at that time. You need be aware of this particularly because many of your nursing clients will be in circumstances or states-of-being where they cannot tolerate or accept your feelings. In these cases—Hold Thy Tongue!

2. The other person is not available and will not be for some time. If J. was going away for the weekend, leaving directly from class, you would not be able to express yourself immediately. Nonavailability also occurs when the person who elicited the feeling is dead. Much time in psychotherapy is devoted to working through feelings regarding deceased parents and other loved/hated persons. It is also possible that the object of a feeling is a massive system that you cannot confront directly, for example, the government or the telephone company.

3. The circumstances are such that direct expression of a feeling could result in harm or injury to yourself. Suppose that J. comes home waving a Big Stick and approaches you menacingly. It would be foolish for you to pick this moment to state your irritation. You will need to cool it for the time being. This applies also to situations, however unlikely, when another person (robber or attacker) might be provoked to further violence against you if you directly express your feelings. You would need to evaluate carefully whether or not to express yourself.

However, these described times do not negate your experience of feelings, and you will need to formulate some interventions for yourself when it is not wise or possible to externalize the feelings through direct expression. Examples of these are physical activity (jogging, swimming, using a punching bag) and stating your feelings to a trusted, other person (friend, confidant, counselor). It is essential that you realize that feelings need to be expressed or they can do you harm. Only by externalizing feelings in some way can you fully experience them and then let them go. Until you do get feelings out, they will be unwanted and unneeded "baggage" you carry with you and will probably impede your experience of living.

You likely found this last section somewhat long and "heavy." Take a few minutes, draw some deep breaths and allow your mind to rest. Do not be gone too long though.

Now that you are refreshed, do the following review exercises.

1. List four ways feelings are handled.

a.

b.

c.

d.

2. Write the four steps in the process of handling feelings positively.

a.

b.

c.

d.

3. Briefly describe three circumstances when it would be unsafe, impossible, or inappropriate to express feelings directly.

a.

b.

c.

ANSWERS

1. Four ways feelings are handled.

a. obliquely—indirectly

b. denial—internalization

c. "acting out"—displacement

d. taking responsibility and fully experiencing them

2. Positive (healthy) handling of feelings.

a. identifying the feeling

b. labeling and describing

c. expressing and externalizing

d. accepting responsibility and expression

3. Circumstances that preclude direct expression of feelings.

a. The other person cannot or will not accept expression of feelings.

b. The other person (or object of feeling) is not available.

c. Direct expression could result in harm to self.

Identify at least one way by which you, yourself, deal with (or could resolve) unexpressed feeling(s).

I handle unexpressed feelings by:

Is this way healthy for you? If not, can you think of more positive "interventions" for working through feelings not fully experienced or expressed?

> Variety's the very spice of life,
> That gives it all its flavor. *COWPER*

With what you have completed thus far, you should be able to differentiate thoughts and feelings. Write a brief description of the difference(s) between these two concepts. No answer will be provided. If you have difficulty describing distinguishing aspects, you need to review what has been covered.

Thoughts are:

Feelings are:

Thoughts and feelings are different in that:

In actuality, the separation of these two notions is artificial; they are both very much a part of the "human condition" experience. If either becomes too strong an influence on functioning, and the other is suppressed or denied, the person can suffer greatly. There is a time and place for each. For example, Luft describes the *naturalist*, a type of leader who relies on thoughts and thinking:

> As a leader, consultant, teacher, or healer, the naturalist is essentially realistic, factual, and impersonal. He wants to find out what the problem is and go to work on it directly . . . . Feelings are simply not important to the naturalist-leader and any undue display of emotion is frowned upon. Reason is the mode; facts count . . . . His own personality is kept out of the picture to the point where he may be criticized for being cold and impersonal (Luft, 1969, pp. 102-103).

When this person is "leading," this attitude may work very well for him/her. You will encounter many times in your nursing career when the naturalist-style of leadership is required, for example, in crisis situations. However, there must also be activity and behavior built-in to living to allow for expression of feelings.

On the other hand, too much feeling can interfere with problem-solving and growth. The individual who is overly influenced by emotions, sensations, and tensions is often impulsive and hysterical-like in behavior. Have you known such people? Are you like that yourself? How would you deal with a coworker or subordinate who displayed this pattern of functioning? There is no easy answer, but you will be ahead of the game if you begin thinking about this problem now.

> Order is the sanity of the mind, the health of the body, the peace of the city, the security of the state. As the beams to a house, as the bones to the microcosm of man, so is order to all things.
>
> *SOUTHEY*

Thoughts and/or feelings are the source of behavior; behavior is the result of these two activities. Either thoughts or feelings can originate the process ending in behavior. That is, any of the following four are possible:

1. thoughts eliciting feelings giving rise to behavior
2. thoughts alone stimulating behavior
3. feelings causing thoughts, which then evoke behavior
4. feelings alone resulting in behavior.

Ideally then, the "order" (from the quote) in your own life can be enhanced by healthy assimilation of all modes of experience. Integration of your own thoughts, feelings and behavior will result in:

1. constructive thinking and dealing with life's problems in a level-headed manner
2. positive experience of emotion, sensations, and tensions with subsequent expression and resolution
3. productive and goal-directed activity.

It is hopefully obvious by now that this "order" of thoughts, feelings and behavior will assist you in living a rich, full life. Of equal importance, it will support your being effective and meaningful in working with clients and others in nursing.

Man know thyself! All wisdom centers there. *YOUNG*

As a Big Wrap-Up to this module, describe your thoughts, feelings, and behavior in reaction to the following situations. You need not write these responses, but give a fair amount of time and attention to each.

1. In the last semester of your nursing program, you experience an overwhelming amount of stress—your lover walks out, a dear friend dies in a car accident, and so on. A consequence of all this is that you fail two out of the four courses you are taking. When the stress subsides, and the dust settles, you reconnoiter to complete the program. After much discussion, you are informed by the director that

you will be allowed to finish on the condition that you repeat the entire semester—including the courses that you passed. (Remember this situation is only hypothetical.)

My thoughts about this situation would be:____________________.

My feelings would be:____________________.

My behavior would be:____________________.

2. After a week of being the "team leader," you have lunch with a coworker. It has been very hectic on the unit, with many crisis-type events, and you feel good that you ran things fairly smoothly and efficiently. You state to your meal companion, "I'm a little relieved this week is over." That person responds, "I can understand that. I guess you just aren't cut out to be a leader."

My thoughts would be:____________________.

My feelings would be:____________________.

My behavior would be:____________________.

3. After a period of arduous study, you are now finished with this module, and are thanked for your attention and participation. You are instructed to complete the posttest and check your answers.

My thoughts are:____________________.

My feelings are:____________________.

My behavior will be:____________________.

Think, feel and behave in good health!

Posttest

1. Define *thoughts.* Thoughts are:

2. Fill in the blanks. (A)__________________ are the result of using the mind to reason based on a (B)__________________ for growth and development present at birth. Thinking (C)__________________ (is, is not) directly observable, and actualization depends on the (D)__________________ between the individual and (E)__________________

3. Briefly describe three mental activities directly related to thinking.

   A.

   B.

   C.

4. Define *feelings.* Feelings are:

5. List three kinds of feelings.

   A.

   B.

   C.

6. Write five physiological effects or manifestations of the experience of feelings.

   A. D.

   B. E.

   C.

7. List four methods of dealing with feelings.

   A.

   B.

   C.

   D.

8. Write the four steps in the process of handling feelings positively.

   A.

   B.

   C.

   D.

9. Describe three situations in which you would choose not to express feelings directly.

   A.

   B.

   C.

10. Complete the following sentence. Thoughts and feelings are different in that:

11. Briefly describe the relatedness of thoughts, feelings, and behavior.

12. List three benefits of integrating your thoughts, feelings, and behavior.

    A.

    B.

    C.

Posttest Answers

1. Thoughts are the direct result of thinking or using the power of reasoning; a collection of ideas or concepts; the object of attention or consideration.
2. A. thoughts
   B. potential
   C. is not
   D. interaction
   E.. environmental factors
3. A. "mind's eye"—fantasies, images, needs, or desires.
   B. attitude development—habits of thought
   C. learning—problem solving
4. Feelings are the result of touch or physical sensation; awareness of sensation, emotions and sensitivities; tension of need states.
5. A. emotion
   B. physical sensations
   C. tension of need states
6. A. muscle tension
   B. changes in blood pressure
   C. distribution of blood between body interior and surface
   D. alteration of heart rate
   E. alteration in persperation
   or: changes in respiration—pupil changes—change in gastrointestinal motility—galvanic skin response
7. A. indirectly—obliquely
   B. denial—internalization
   C. displacement—acting out
   D. taking responsibility and experiencing them
8. A. identifying feeling
   B. labeling and describing feeling
   C. expressing and externalizing feeling
   D. accepting responsibility and expression
9. A. The other person cannot or will not accept direct expression.
   B. Object of feeling is not available.
   C. Direct expression might result in harm to self.

10. Thoughts and feelings are different in that the former involve the intellect and the mind, while the latter have their origin in the body and physical awareness (or any similar explanation).
11. Behavior is the result or expression of thoughts and/or feelings. Behavior can originate in thoughts, in feelings, or in both, that is, thoughts-feelings-behavior, feelings-thoughts-behavior, thought-behavior, or feelings-behavior.
12. A. constructive thinking and problem-solving.
    B. positive and full experience of feelings
    C. productive and goal-directed behavior

REFERENCES

1. Burgess, Ann W., and Aaron Lazare. "Feelings, Thoughts, and Behaviors," in *Psychiatric Nursing in the Hospital and the Community*, 2nd ed. (Englewood Cliffs, New Jersey: Prentice-Hall, Inc., 1976), pp. 203-211.

2. Luft, Joseph. *Of Human Interaction* (Palo Alto, California: Mayfield Publishing Company, 1969).

3. Poland, Ronal G. *Human Experience: A Psychology of Growth* (St. Louis: C. V. Mosby Company, 1974).

4. Travelbee, Joyce. *Intervention in Psychiatric Nursing* (Philadelphia: F. A. Davis Company, 1969), pp. 124-175.

5. *Webster's New World Dictionary of the American Language* (New York: Popular Library, 1975).

Self-Disclosure

DIRECTIONS

1. Complete the pretest. If you answer all the questions correctly, you may choose to complete the unit on self-disclosure for added enrichment and knowledge.

2. After the pretest, complete the activities as directed. The activities and exercises should be completed in the order presented.

3. In order to complete the unit, you will need a pencil or pen. No other materials are needed.

4. A posttest will be given at the end of the unit. Successful completion of this test is necessary for you to have met the unit objectives.

OBJECTIVES Upon completion of this unit on self-disclosure, the learner will be able to:

1. Define self-disclosure.
2. Describe two related concepts: self-awareness and self-acceptance.
3. Explain four positive results of high-level self-awareness.
4. Identify four areas of living directly influenced by self-awareness.
5. List three methods of developing self-awareness.
6. Restate four positive results of self-acceptance.
7. Identify at least one personal strength and describe how it can be utilized to develop self-acceptance.
8. Discuss four positive results of self-disclosure.
9. Differentiate appropriate and inappropriate disclosing of self.
10. Formulate a plan for practicing self-disclosure in interpersonal relationships.

Pretest

True (T) or False (F).

1. Self-disclosure is the act of making yourself manifest.
2. Self-disclosure means revealing intimate details of your past life.
3. Self-awareness will help you to recognize your strengths and ignore your limitations.
4. Being highly critical of yourself will assist you in developing self-acceptance.
5. You should forget your own philosophy of living and set of values when giving patient-centered nursing care.
6. The "self" of an individual is constantly in a state of flux and change.
7. You should use your potentials as consistently as possible.
8. Anxiety and frustration are seldom sources of positive growth.
9. Introspection and "soul searching" can assist you in being self-aware.
10. Contemplation of your physical state can enhance self-awareness.
11. A self-accepting individual is inclined to resist efforts of others to dominate him or her.

12. People who accept themselves can restrict their enjoyment to a few selected activities.

13. All people have solid strengths that are unidentified and unused.

14. Modesty about your positive attributes is a strength in itself.

15. Self-disclosure will help you to avoid experiencing rejection.

16. Personal responsibility is a direct result of disclosing yourself in communication.

17. Self-disclosure is appropriate even if it is not reciprocated.

18. A crisis in a relationship often speeds up self-disclosure.

19. You should self-disclose regardless of the effect it will have on others.

20. Self-disclosure involves risk taking, and should be coercive.

Pretest Answers

1. True	2. False	3. False	4. False	5. False	6. True
7. True	8. False	9. True	10. True	11. True	12. False
13. True	14. False	15. False	16. True	17. False	
18. True	19. False	20. False			

INTRODUCTION

This above all: To thine own self be true;
And it must follow, as the night the day,
Thou cans't not then be false to any man. *SHAKESPEARE*

A major objective in life is that the person will assume individual responsibility:

1. for interactive process by communicating reactions to others
2. for self by setting limits on own involvement and verbally communicating this to others
3. for own ideas, feelings, perceptions, and behaviors.

This goal emphasizes the importance of your learning how to share with others and to accept personal responsibility for what you share. To do this effectively, you need to know yourself, like yourself, and reveal yourself to some degree; thus, self-awareness, self-acceptance, and self-disclosure. Very importantly, having these in your grasp will aid you in your nursing practice and entire career.

For clarification, this presentation will separate self-awareness, self-acceptance, and self-disclosure. You need to keep in mind, though, that the division is artificial, and done only for elucidation of the concepts. In actuality, all three ideas are part and parcel of the same thing—interpersonal sharing and relating.

SELF AWARENESS

The most difficult thing in life is to know yourself. *THALES*

Man know thyself! All wisdom centers there. *YOUNG*

Based on the above quotes, you can see that self-awareness is simply knowledge of yourself—knowing who, what, where, how, and why you are. People commonly believe that they possess this knowledge. This may be true to an extent, but you should always strive to increase your level of self-awareness. High-level self-awareness is an invaluable aid in living a rich, full life.

What can self-awareness do for you? For one thing, it can assist you in recognizing your own strengths *and* limitations. When deciding on a goal towards which to strive, you need to evaluate your ability to succeed. For example, if, when you decided to become a nurse, you had been aware of a gross deficiency in the physical sciences, you would have needed to overcome this limitation. Or you might have revised your goal. In any case, being *aware* of part of your *self* would have helped you in making a decision about your life.

Self-awareness can also get you "in touch" with your philosophy of living and set of values. This will be the very basis of your functioning—both as a person and as a nurse. Undoubtedly during your career, you will encounter situations where your values are tested, for example, a Catholic nurse being asked to participate in an abortion. What will you do? How will you handle it so that your patients receive needed care and yet your philosophy is not compromised? Self-awareness is the first step towards answering these questions.

Self-confidence and being comfortable with your self-image can result from knowing yourself. These traits are essential for your continued, positive growth and development. Along with this, unceasing expanding of your self-knowledge would serve to emphasize the existential fact that you are always "becoming." Your self never "is," but is in a constant state of flux and change; thus, "becoming."

In review, four positive results of high level self-awareness are:

1. recognizing your strengths *and* limitations
2. knowing your set of values and philosophy of living
3. self-confidence and comfort with self-image
4. allowing yourself to grow and "become."

O'Brien has described specific areas of living directly influenced by self-awareness (1974, pp. 58-64). These areas are ones each of us must deal with, with a certain amount of success. First, you need to identify your *potentials*, be willing to use them to the best of your ability as consistently as possible, and accept them as valuable aids to your growth. Second, you need to be aware of your own unique *anxieties,* and utilize them as sources of positive growth. Third, when your efforts do not produce the results you would like, *frustrations* will rear their ugly heads and you must manage them and not allow them to inhibit your capability. Last, you will surely meet with *conflicts* that are either a strife for mastery, a hostile encounter, or a prolonged mental or moral struggle between incompatible desires or aims. These contentions, if handled adequately, can produce strength and resiliency for future resource.

List four areas of living directly influenced by self-awareness.

1.	3.
2.	4.

How does one develop self-awareness? One easy method is *introspection* or "soul searching." To try this out, think of a person you dislike, and answer the following questions:

1. What about this person do I dislike?
2. What does this person do that I dislike?
3. What irritating differences exist between this person and myself?
4. Does this person remind me of someone I have known that I also disliked?
5. Does this person inhibit my strengths?
6. Does this person challenge my values or philosophy?
7. Does this person threaten my self-confidence or self-image?
8. Does this person block my "becoming"?
9. In what ways does this person spark in me anxiety, frustration, and conflict?
10. What can I do about this person and the dislike I feel?

Although briefly presented, this process should be carried out slowly and thoughtfully. You can easily do the same thing about something you *like*—a person, a song, a book and so on.

Another simple way to increase self-awareness is *reflection* on your physical state of being—body awareness. Sit quietly for a few minutes and consider each part of your body, from toe to head. Think of the following questions:

1. What is my general feeling state? Tired? Tense? Relaxed?
2. Where in my body do I feel pain or discomfort?

3. Where do I feel tension? Relaxation?

4. Are there external causes for my body state? The chair? Lighting? Temperature of the room?

5. Are there external events affecting my body state? Noise? People talking? Someone walking by?

6. What can I do to improve my feeling state? Taking some deep breaths? Walking around for a while? Alternately tensing and relaxing different parts of my body?

Caution: Do not get too relaxed! A certain amount of tension is necessary for you to continue with this module.

There are also *structured exercises* that will increase your level of self-awareness. The following, having to do with values clarification, is an example. Read the story, and follow the instructions.

Five people took a cruise. The five people were: A, B, C, D, and E. A and B were in love, and planned to marry the next week. A storm came up and the boat was tossed and battered. It hit a rock and capsized between two islands. A, C, and D managed to swim to one island; B and E made it to the other.

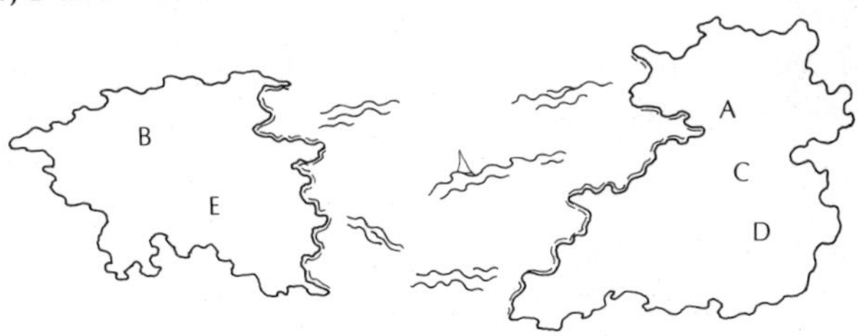

A and B were separated, and A was heartbroken. A wanted to get to B as soon as possible. But there was a problem. Sharks! (Shades of *Jaws.*) The water between the islands was full of them. But A was determined to reach B some way. A loved B and felt a need to be together.

A got an idea: C or D could help build a raft and sail across to B. A went to C, and asked for help. C studied the problem, and finally said, "The odds are against it. If we did build a raft, the materials wouldn't hold up. Besides it's so windy, and the ocean is so rough, that it just isn't feasible. No, I'm sorry, but it's too risky." So A went to D. D looked A in the eye, and said, "Yes. For a price." A was stunned, said, "Never!" and ran away.

Finally it became unbearable. A just could not live without B any longer and so gave in to D. They built a raft, and somehow managed to reach the other island.

A was very happy, and ran straight to B. But B pushed A away, and said, "I know how you got over here. I don't want anything to do with you." A dissolved in tears, crying, "I only did it for you. I wanted to be with you. Can't you understand that?" But B was steadfast. Meanwhile, E, overhearing all this, thought B was a jerk. E went to A and said, "Anyone who would go through all that for the love of another person must be pretty special. If you will have me A, I'd be glad to marry you."

Okay, you have read the story. Now, list the characters in the order you prefer them. In other words, rate the people in order, from the person you respect most to the one you respect least.

1. 2. 3. 4. 5.

Two different interpretations of what each character symbolizes appear below.

Character	Interpretation #1	Interpretation #2
A	love	sex
B	morals	morality
C	education	business-like
D	sex	power
E	family	security

Using whichever interpretation seems more logical to you, list your own hierarchy of values, as indicated by your above choices.

1.

2.

3.

4.

5.

The reliability of the interpretations will not be argued here. For the present, accept them as valid. Did your hierarchy surprise you? If you had been given the words, would you have put them in the same order? Did this exercise increase your self-awareness? The results will be referred to later, so keep them in mind.

List three means of developing self-awareness.

1.

2.

3.

SELF-ACCEPTANCE

The reverence of a man's self is, next religion,
the chiefest bridle of all vices. *LORD BACON*

"Self-acceptance is a high regard for yourself, or, conversely, a lack of cynicism about your self" (Johnson, 1972, p. 142). Generally, a high level of self-acceptance is reflected in a high quality of personal adjustment. An individual's mental health depends, to a great extent, on the quality of his/her feelings about him or herself. Satir has a unique way of looking at feelings of self-worth, which she calls "pot" (1972). If a person is feeling high self-acceptance, the person is experiencing "high pot." Low level self-esteem indicates "low pot." A mental exercise Satir suggests will be presented here (Satir, 1972, pp. 23-24).

Can you remember some time recently when your spirits were up? Perhaps you were told that you had been promoted; or you wore new clothes and received several compliments; or you handled a difficult problem and everything turned out well. Try to go back now and feel again the feelings you had then. That is what it is like to feel "high pot."

Can you remember another occasion, when you made an embarrassing slip, or a costly error, or you were scolded angrily by someone; or you felt helpless in handling a problem? Again, go back and relive the feelings you had, even though it is painful. That is what it is like to feel "low pot."

Now relax for a moment, then feel the state of your "pot" today. Is it high or low? Has something special happened to give you this feeling, or do you feel this way most of the time?

The above activity should have helped you expand self-awareness of your self-acceptance. Did it? Satir's book is strongly recommended as an easy to read, stimulating work on communication and growth and development.

Self-acceptance is obviously in your favor, but what are some of the specific benefits to be derived from high-level self-esteem? These include:

1. Seeing yourself as liked, wanted, acceptable to others, capable and worthy—in short, a nice person

2. Seeing the world as a congenial place in which to live, work, and love

3. Increased potential for growth, happiness, and good relationships

4. Increased acceptance of others, and ability to be supportive of yourself and others

Regarding item 4, there is a saying, "You are what you hate." This means simply that we often feel negatively about someone or something because an unacceptable or undesirable piece of ourselves is reflected. With this in mind, it is easy to see that as we accept ourselves more, we will be able to accept others more too. Can you identify something you dislike in others that is a mirror of part of you? Be honest with yourself—you have nothing to lose, and much to gain.

For further clarification, slowly and carefully read Johnson's (1972) "Characteristics of Self-Accepting Individuals" listed below. People who have a strong self-accepting attitude present the following behavorial picture:

1. They believe strongly in certain values and principles and are willing to defend them even in the face of strong group opinion. However, they feel personally secure enough to modify them if new experience and evidence suggest they are in error.

2. They are capable of acting on their own judgment without feeling excessively guilty or regretful if others disapprove of what they have done.

3. They do not spend undue time worrying about what is coming tomorrow, what has happened in the past, or what is taking place in the present.

4. They have confidence in their ability to deal with problems, even in the face of failure and setbacks.

5. They feel equal to others as a person, not superior or inferior, irrespective of the differences in specific abilities, family backgrounds, or attitudes of others toward them.

6. They are able to take for granted that they are persons of interest and value to others, at least to those with whom they choose to associate.

7. They can accept praise without the pretense of false modesty and compliments without feeling guilty.

8. They are inclined to resist the efforts of others to dominate them.

9. They are able to accept the idea and admit to others that they are capable of feeling a wide range of impulses and desires, ranging from being angry to being loving, from being sad to being happy, from feeling deep resentment to feeling deep acceptance.

10. They are able to genuinely enjoy themselves in a wide variety of activities involving work, play, creative self-expression, companionship, or loafing.

11. They are sensitive to the needs of others, to accepted social customs, and particularly to the idea that they cannot enjoy themselves at the expense of others (Johnson, 1972, pp. 144-145).

One way to build self-acceptance is to increase your awareness of strengths. We all have different strengths; and all have solid strengths that are presently unidentified and unused. An activity, suggested by Johnson's writing, can help you identify at least one personal strength (1972, pp. 145-148). As Johnson states: (1972, p. 145)

> Through identification of these strengths we may increase our ability to relate to other people. The word *strength* refers to any skill, talent, ability, or personal trait which helps you to function more productively. Through identifying your personal strengths you may increase your regard for yourself and, therefore, increase your self-acceptance. In addition, you may explore and develop your potential strengths into solid strengths, you may intensify your presently known strengths by practicing them, and you may restructure weaknesses into strengths.

This is no place for modesty. An inferiority attitude or the unwillingness to be open about your positive attributes is not a strength. You are not being asked to brag, only to be realistic and open about the strengths that you possess. The procedure for the exercise is as follows:

1. Think of the things you do well, things which you are proud of having done, things for which you feel a sense of accomplishment. Briefly list three positive accomplishments, or successes, of the past. Be as specific as you can. Three of my positive accomplishments are:

2. Examine your successes and identify the strengths you utilized to achieve them. My personal strengths are:

3. After you have identified your strengths, ask yourself, "What might be keeping me from utilizing all my strengths?" The barriers to my utilizing my strengths are:

4. Think about your successes and strengths. How may your strengths be utilized to improve the number or quality of your close relationships? Set a goal for the next week concerning how you might improve either the number or the quality of your close relationships. Plan how utilization of your strengths will help you accomplish this goal. My goal is:

My strengths involved are:

The ways I will utilize my strengths to accomplish my goal are:

I will know that my goal is accomplished when:

Another activity will be expressing acceptance to another—one who disagrees with you. Refer back to the hierarchy of values you formulated after the story of A, B, C, D, and E. List them in *reverse* order.

1.
2.
3.
4.
5.

Now, imagine that this list is another person's hierarchy of values, and this person says to you, "My priority is more correct than yours." Write a brief response to this person that would convey acceptance of the different hierarchy without changing yours.

Yes, I can see that our priorities are different. I:

SELF-DISCLOSURE

To conceal anything from those to whom
I am attached, is not in my nature.
I can never close my lips where I
have opened my heart. *DICKENS*

According to Jourard, "Self-disclosure is the act of making yourself manifest, showing yourself so others can perceive you" (1971, p. 19). Or, as Johnson states (1972, p. 10):

> *Self-disclosure* may be defined as revealing how you are reacting to the present situation and giving any information about the past that is relevant to understanding how you are reacting to the present.

Your reactions to people and events are not facts as much as feelings. To be self-disclosing means to share with another person how you feel about something the person has done or said, or how you feel about events that have just occurred. It does not mean revealing intimate details of your past life. Making personal "confessions" about your past may lead to a temporary intimacy, but a relationship is built by stating your reactions to events you both experience or to what the other person says or does. A person comes to really know and understand you not through getting your past history, but through knowing how you react. Past history is helpful only if it clarifies why you are reacting in a certain way. Egan has a particularly good outline and discussion of self-disclosure; you are encouraged to study it (1970).

Based on the information given, write your own definition of self-disclosure. Self-disclosure is:

What does self-disclosure do for you? Why should you take the risk of exposing your feelings, and maybe being rejected or hurt? One positive result of disclosing yourself is increased levels of self-awareness and self-acceptance. Another payoff is that you will form closer relationships because people will come to truly know you, thereby meeting a basic human need of yours. This does not mean that you will never experience rejection. However, if people accept *or* reject you as you really are, you can relinquish the "roles" that are dishonest representations of your self. You will be able to put your energy into being the person you want to be, and be intimate and close with whom you wish. At the risk of giving advice—do not waste your energy on people who openly reject you. Consider it their problem; after all, it is their loss.

To further help you form closer relationships, self-disclosure will encourage others to reveal more of themselves to you. Thus, you will get to know them better. Along with this, sharing feelings and reactions will aid you to be accepting of others while perhaps disagreeing with or disapproving of the way they behave. This is important in nursing where you will encounter many clients doing things that you cannot accept, for example, a parent "battering" a child.

A definite benefit of self-disclosure is that as you open yourself more, you will gain an increased sense of personal responsibility. Refer back to the objective described at the beginning of this presentation. As a maturing adult, it is essential that you accept the responsibility for what you feel, think, and do, and also, for the consequences of your feelings, thoughts, and behavior. This will increase your self-direction and give you more determination of your activities. A negative example of this is the individual who attributes his or her "lot in life" to everything external and everyone else. Have you met such a person? What was your reaction?

Which of the following are *not* positive results of self-disclosure?

1. Increased self-awareness and self-acceptance
2. People will know you better
3. People will reject you more
4. Others will self-disclose more
5. You will agree with everyone
6. You will reject others more
7. Increased personal responsibility

Items 3, 5, and 6 are not positive results of self-disclosure. If your responses were incorrect, review the previous information.

To expound on the appropriateness of self-disclosure, consider the following by Johnson (1972):

> Self-disclosure must be relevant to your relationship with the other person and appropriate to the situation you are in. You can be too self-disclosing. A person who reveals too much of his reactions too fast may scare others away; a relationship is built gradually except in rare and special cases . . . . Self-disclosure is appropriate when:
>
> 1. It is *not* a random or isolated act but rather is part of an ongoing relationship.
> 2. It is reciprocated.
> 3. It concerns what is going on within and between persons in the present.
> 4. It creates a reasonable chance of improving the relationship.
> 5. It is speeded up in a crisis in the relationship.
> 6. It gradually moves to a deeper level.
>
> While relationships are built through self-disclosure, there are times when you will want to hide your reactions to the present situation

from another person. If people have clearly shown themselves to be untrustworthy, it is foolish to be self-disclosing with them. If you know from past experiences that the other person will misinterpret or overreact to your self-disclosure, you may wish to keep silent.

Another activity suggested by Johnson, which focuses on your interpersonal patterns or interaction with other individuals, will be presented here (1972, pp.34-35). It will help you think about how you behave when you initiate a relationship or how you act in a group. The procedure for the exercise is as follows:

1. Fill out the verb checklist below. The twenty verbs listed describe some of the ways people feel and act from time to time. Think of your behavior in interaction with other people. How do you feel and act with other people? Check the five verbs that best describe your behavior in interaction with others as you see it.

2. Analyze the meaning of the verbs you checked by following the instructions, which are found following the checklist.

3. Share the results of the exercise with someone you know, and ask for his/her comments on whether they perceive you similarly or differently than the results of this activity indicate.

acquiesces	disapproves
advises	evades
agrees	initiates
analyzes	judges
assists	leads
concedes	obliges
cooperates	relinquishes
coordinates	resists
criticizes	retreats
directs	withdraws

There are two underlying factors or traits involved in the list of verbs: dominance (authority or control) and sociability (intimacy or friendliness).

Most people tend to like to control things (high dominance) or let others control things (low dominance). Similarly most people tend to be very warm and personal (high sociability) or to be somewhat cold and impersonal (low sociability), In the following boxes, circle the five verbs you used to describe yourself. The set in which three or more verbs are circled represents your *interpersonal pattern tendency.*

	High dominance	Low dominance
High sociability	advises coordinates directs initiates leads	acquiesces agrees assists cooperates obliges
Low sociability	analyzes criticizes disapproves judges resists	concedes evades relinquishes retreats withdraws

For another activity, share the story presented earlier (island conflict) with someone you interact with regularly. It may be someone you are intimate with, or someone you feel close to in a relationship. Whomever you select, have this person complete the activity, then share your results with the person. Are they similar or grossly different? What does each of these mean in your relationship? Can you accept the differences? Can the other person? Share your feelings and reactions with the other person, and encourage her/him to do the same. When you have time, share the story exercise with other people you know.

As a summary, consider the following points, which will increase the chances that self-disclosure will improve a relationship, that is, "Constructive Self-Disclosure" (Johnson, 1972, pp. 36-39).

1. Self-disclosure must begin with a desire to improve your relationship with the other person.

2. Try to create a shared understanding of your relationship.

3. Realize that self-disclosure involves risk-taking.

4. Although the discussion may become intense, spirited, angry, or tearful, it should be noncoercive and should not be an attempt to make the other person change.

5. Timing is important. Reactions should be shared at a time as close as possible to the behavior that aroused them so that both persons will know exactly what behavior is being discussed.

6. Disturbing situations should be discussed as they happen; hurt feelings and annoyances should not be saved up and dropped on another person all at one time.

7. Paraphrase the other person's comments about you to make sure you understand them as the person means them.

8. Statements are more helpful if they are specific rather than general, tentative rather than absolute, and informing rather than ordering.

9. Use perception-checking responses to insure that you are not making false assumptions about the other's feelings.

10. The least helpful kinds of statements are those that sound as if they are information about the other person, but are really expressions of your own feelings, for example, judgments, name-calling, accusations, commands, and sarcasm.

11. The most helpful kinds of information about yourself and your reactions are behavior descriptions and descriptions of your own feelings.

You have now completed the module. Complete the posttest, and check your answers. Thank you for your attention and participation. Self-disclosure will serve you well—make the most of it!

Posttest

Circle the correct answer.

1. Which of the following is the *best* definition of self-disclosure?

   A. the act of revealing the intimate details of your past life
   B. the act of making yourself manifest, showing yourself so others can reject you
   C. revealing how you are reacting to the present and giving relevant information about the past
   D. revealing yourself and your feelings at all times in all relationships

2. Which of the following statements is *not* true of self-awareness?

   A. Self-awareness is knowing who, what, where, how and why you are.
   B. By adulthood, there is little need to increase your self-awareness.
   C. People often believe they possess adequate self-awareness.
   D. High level self-awareness is valuable in living a full and happy life.

3. All of the following are positive results of high-level self-awareness except:

   A. recognizing your strengths and ignoring limitations
   B. knowing your set of values and philosophy of living
   C. self-confidence and liking your self-image
   D. allowing yourself to grow and change as needed

4. Which of the following is *not* an area of living positively influenced by self-awareness?

   A. potentials
   B. conceits
   C. frustrations
   D. anxieties
   E. conflicts

5. All of the following are methods of developing self-awareness *except*:

   A. introspection
   B. structured activity
   C. rationalization
   D. reflection

6. Which of the following statements is *not* true of self-acceptance?

   A. Amount of self-acceptance is mirrored in the quality of personal adjustment.
   B. Satir's "pot" is synonymous with level of self-acceptance or self-esteem.
   C. An individual's mental health depends on his or her feelings about him or herself.
   D. Self-acceptance indicates cynicism about yourself and high self-regard.

7. Which of the following is a *positive* result of self-acceptance?

   A. seeing yourself as an "okay" person
   B. decreased potential for good relationships
   C. seeing the world as an unfriendly place
   D. decreased acceptance of others

8. All of the following are true of personal strengths *except*:

   A. Everyone has strengths that are unidentified and unused.
   B. Strength refers to any skill that helps you function productively.
   C. By identifying strengths, you may restructure your limitations.
   D. Being closed about your positive attributes is a strength in itself.

9. Which of the following is *not* a positive result of self-disclosure?

   A. You will agree with everyone.
   B. Increased personal responsibility.
   C. People will know you better.
   D. Others will self-disclose more.
   E. Increased self-awareness and self-acceptance

10. All the following are principles of *appropriate* self-disclosure *except* (more than one answer):

    A. It is reciprocated.
    B. It is a random or isolated act.
    C. No account is taken of the effect it will have on the other person.
    D. It is not speeded up in a crisis in the relationship.
    E. It creates a chance of improving the relationship.
    F. It gradually moves to a deeper level.
    G. It concerns what is going on within and between persons in the present.

Posttest Answers

1. C	2. B	3. A	4. B	5. C	6. D	7. A	8. D
9. A	10. B, C, D						

REFERENCES

1. Egan, Gerard. *Encounter: Group Processes for Interpersonal Growth* (Belmont, California: Brooks, Cole Publishing Co., 1970), pp. 190-245.

2. Johnson, David W. *Reaching Out: Interpersonal Effectiveness and Self Actualization* (Englewood Cliffs, New Jersey: Prentice-Hall, Inc., 1972), pp. 9-14, 141-150.

3. Jourard, Sidney M. *The Transparent Self* (New York: D. Van Nostrand Co., 1971).

4. O'Brien, Maureen J. *Communications and Relationships in Nursing* (St. Louis: C. V. Mosby Co., 1974), pp. 56-64.

5. Satir, Virginia. *Peoplemaking* (Palo Alto, California: Science and Behavior Books, Inc., 1972), pp. 20-29.

Trust

DIRECTIONS

1. Complete the pretest. If you answer all the questions correctly, you may choose to complete the unit on trust for added enrichment and knowledge.

2. After the pretest, complete the activities as directed. The activities and exercises should be completed in the order presented.

3. In order to complete the unit, you will need a pencil or pen. No other materials are needed.

4. A posttest will be given at the end of the unit. Successful completion of this test is necessary for you to have met the unit objectives.

OBJECTIVES

Upon completion of this unit on trust, the learner will be able to:

1. State a working definition of trust.

2. Identify the qualities of a person who has trust for self and others.

3. State three elements of communication that make trust possible.

4. Describe two ways to determine if self-disclosure is appropriate in a relationship.

5. State the term most commonly confused with trust.

6. Describe the two most common issues related to trust in the nurse-client relationship.

7. List the three questions we deal with when we enter a new group.

8. State the two major facets of risk in a group.

Pretest

1. The current definition of trust is to:

   A. console
   B. rely upon
   C. comfort
   D. be dependable

2. All of the following characteristics are typical of one who trusts *except*:

   A. comfortable with an increased awareness of self
   B. able to share self-awareness with anyone
   C. accepts new experiences
   D. demonstrates consistency between words and actions

3. Trust is possible when verbal and nonverbal communication are:

   A. honest, practical, relevant
   B. clear, consistent, congruent
   C. holistic, efficient, valid
   D. concise, metacommunicative, timely

4. We usually disclose too much because we:

   A. misread the metacommunication in the relationship.
   B. are involved in a reciprocal relationship.
   C. assume too much responsibility for the relationship.
   D. incorrectly assess the depth of the relationship.

5. In a crisis, self-disclosure is more:

   A. difficult
   B. spontaneous
   C. rapid
   D. controlled

6. The most common abuse of the term *to trust* is to confuse it with to

   A. confide
   B. rely upon
   C. accept
   D. tolerate

7. When a client sends a verbal message to a nurse he or she expects the nurse to hear the report and the:

   A. communication
   B. content
   C. context
   D. command

8. A common problem that occurs in relationship to trust, in the nurse-client relationship, is when the client asks the nurse to:

   A. discuss a personal matter
   B. tell him or her what his or her temperature is
   C. give him or her a pain medication
   D. keep a secret

9. When we form a new group we have to immediately deal with all of the following questions *except:*

   A. Is there a trusting atmosphere?
   B. Who has the power?
   C. Who is involved?
   D. How close can we get?

10. As trust develops in a group, risk is:

    A. ventured
    B. lessened
    C. greater
    D. the same

Pretest Answers

1. B	2. B	3. B	4. D	5. C	6. D	7. D
8. D	9. A	10. B				

INTRODUCTION

Most of us want to trust others and be trusted. How many people do you trust? List them.

1.

2.

3.

4.

5.

If you have listed five names you are very fortunate indeed. Trust, however, means different things for different people at different times. Sometimes we do not feel trust for anyone, while at other times we feel trust for everyone in a large group.

When you look at the index of a book about communication, nursing, psychology, or behavior you will not find very much written specifically about trust. At the same time, as nurses we feel that trust is extremely important in our relationships with others.

This module is designed to assist you in thinking about the concept of trust in relation to yourself, your friends and relatives, your clients, and groups of people.

TRUST—A DEFINITION The word *trust* originally came from the Scandinavian language and meant to comfort, to console, or to confide in. The current definition of trust is *to rely upon.*

Which of the following definitions describes your own understanding of trust?

"Trust is confidence in or reliance on some quality or attitude of a person or thing, or the truth of a statement" (Lederer and Jackson, 1968).

"Trust is a sensing, a feeling, that at least some important sectors of the world are dependable and that some of the people in the world are warm, caring, available, and friendly" (Poland, 1974, pp. 16–17).

"When you rely on someone without question, that is trust" (Lewis, 1973).

"Trust is the expectation of the opportunity to function and to become in a world which provides support and freedom" (Luft, 1969).

Write your preferred definition or one of your own here.

Trust is:

HOW MUCH DO YOU TRUST? Think of a person you trust. Write the name of the person here: ______________________.
Fill in the blanks of the following statements with one of these words: Never—Seldom—Occasionally—Usually—Always (Human Development Institute, 1967).

1. I level with him/her ______________________.
   He/she levels with me ______________________.
2. I make clear what I am saying ______________________.
   He/she makes clear what he/she is saying ______________________.
3. I know the kind of person he/she is ______________________.
   He/she knows the kind of person I am ______________________.
4. I accept him/her for what he/she is ______________________.
   He/she accepts me for what I am ______________________.
5. I feel my ideas are worth expressing ______________________.
   He/she feels his/her ideas are worth expressing ______________________.
6. I risk saying what I feel even when I know he/she may disagree ______________________.
   He/she risks saying what he/she feels even when he/she knows I may disagree ______________________.

Evidence shows that those who trust have the following qualities:

1. comfortable with an increased awareness of self, goals, and motivation
2. able to share self-awareness with appropriate people
3. accept others who deviate from their own ways of thinking, feeling, and acting without feeling an intense need to change them

4. accept new experiences

5. demonstrate a consistency between words and actions that lasts over a period of time

6. able to delay gratification. (Carlson, 1970)

Consider your answers about yourself and your trusted partner and determine how much you trust.

Do you think he or she would agree with your answers? It is a great compliment to be trusted. Why don't you share this activity with the person you trust and discuss the concept of trust in your relationship? Lederer and Jackson (1968), feel that trust is possible when verbal and nonverbal communication is:

1. consistent

2. congruent

3. clear

Make a guess as to which point your trusted partner would say your relationship needs the most improvement in. Ask him or her about this too, if you feel up to that much feedback.

Are you communicating with your clients in a consistent, congruent, and clear manner? Ask a colleague to go with you when you visit a client, then ask for an evaluation of your communication with regard to these three elements of trust.

TRUST AND SELF-DISCLOSURE Think of a situation in which you trusted and thus disclosed yourself to another person. Write out your answers to the following questions:

1. Describe how what you shared was relevant to the relationship.

2. Was the self-disclosure reciprocal? In what way?

3. Was your timing for revealing yourself appropriate?

4. How did the other person validate having received the information you disclosed?

5. Describe the effect of the disclosure on the other person.

6. In what way did revealing yourself create a risk for you?

7. Are you glad or sad that you trusted the person? Explain.

The previous questions are ways of evaluating if you used appropriate self-disclosure in terms of the nature of the relationship. In appropriate trusting relationships, self-disclosure is reciprocal, and the responsibility for the relationship and its depth are shared (Luft, 1969).

We sometimes disclose too much because we do not assess the qualities or depth of different relationships. Generally we disclose ourselves gradually as we develop trust in another person. In times of a crisis, however, we often reveal ourselves more rapidly.

Describe below a situation where you now realize you over-disclosed yourself.

Describe now a situation in which a client trusted you and disclosed something which indicated that trust.

TRUST OR TOLERATION Luft (1969) states that the most common abuse of the term *to trust* is to confuse it with *to tolerate.*

In order to view this problem more clearly, make a list of friends or relatives who tolerate you as you are.

1.

2.

3.

Now make another list of friends or relatives who trust you to *become* in your own way.

1.

2.

3.

Sometimes we become frustrated and angry when we expect trust and receive toleration. What were some of the feelings this activity stirred up within you? Can you show some of them here?

What behavior do you exhibit that may cause people to tolerate rather than trust you?

Is it possible that any of your clients might feel you tolerate rather than trust them? Explain your answer.

TRUST AND THE NURSE-CLIENT RELATIONSHIP Whenever a nurse and client develop a relationship they must define their mutual roles. In any relationship those involved are presented with the following problems (Haley, 1963):

1. What messages, or what kinds of behavior are to take place in the relationship?

2. Who is to control what is to take place in the relationship?

We are all constantly involved in defining our relationships with others and trust is certainly an essential element.

When the client or the nurse, for example, does not want to develop an in-depth relationship, he or she may talk about TV programs and thus define the relationship as neutral.

If the client or the nurse, and hopefully both, feel a sense of trust they will define the relationship as trustworthy by showing something of personal value in their messages and behavior.

The nurse needs to be alert to the messages of the client as he or she will be expected to hear the report of the message as well as the command.

When the client says "I didn't sleep well last night," he or she trusts the nurse to hear that message as the report, and also trusts the nurse to hear the command of "Please do something about it" or "Please think of me as a person who has not rested" or "Do not expect anything of me today."

It becomes obvious that further data must be collected in order to determine what the command is, and if it is relevant to the relationship.

Think of your most recent experience with a client. Please answer the questions about that relationship:

1. Did the messages you exchanged indicate a reasonable level of trust? Explain.
2. What did you do to enhance the trust component of the relationship?
3. How did your behavior and that of the client reflect trust or mistrust?
4. Who controlled what took place in the relationship?
5. How did you feel about being/not being in control?
6. If you cared for the same client again, how would you alter the relationship in terms of trust?

We often assume that the client will trust us because our intent is good. The truth is that whether or not the client trusts us will be greatly affected by our communication and our behavior.

In general there are two issues that come up repeatedly in the nurse-client relationship in regard to trust.

The first issue is that the client expects us to tell the truth, and we should do so. If you find yourself in a situation where you question the wisdom of telling the truth, talk about it with a nurse whose judgment you value before making a decision not to do so. Keep in mind that when you do not verbally tell the truth your nonverbal communication may reveal the truth anyway.

The second issue is that sometimes a client will ask you to keep a secret. It is nearly always unwise to make such a promise. If the client tells you something that is important to her/his care you are then put in the position of either breaking your trust or neglecting her/his health. Sometimes clients even ask for such a promise to test you, knowing full well your responsibility to the health team. Generally it is useful to tell them you can't promise but you are interested in what they have to say. Most clients do eventually tell you what they want to say, and may even trust you more when they know you are reliable.

TRUST IN A GROUP When we enter a new group there are three questions we deal with immediately, although maybe not consciously. The questions are:

1. Who is involved in this group?
2. Who has the power?
3. How close can we get?

Consider these questions in relation to a group of which you are a member. Write out the answers if you wish.

Egan (1971) says there are two facets of risk in a group:

1. risking to expose oneself
2. risking to expose another

When we do take the risk to expose our self or others, and it is successful, we feel strengthened and trusting. When we take the risk and it is successful we then feel less trusting. The more we can take that risk and help others do so, the more a climate of trust is developed in the group. As trust develops, risk is lessened. It is naive to think, however, that trust is constant. Trust varies and is on a continuum according to the circumstances and the situation.

Think about yourself in relation to your group as you circle a yes or no response to the following statements:

1. yes no I feel involved in the group.
2. yes no I have some power in the group.
3. yes no I am as close to others as I want to be.

4. yes no I am not afraid of the group members.
5. yes no I show myself to speak freely.
6. yes no I am my usual self in the group.
7. yes no I do not say different things outside of the group.
8. yes no I have taken the risk to expose myself.
9. yes no I have taken the risk to expose others.
10. yes no I am comfortable with my trust level in the group.

Your reactions will vary, of course, from group to group and even within a particular group. If you have circled some statements "no" it tends to indicate you do not trust yourself or the group.

List three things you can do within the group to strengthen the level of trust for yourself and others.

1.
2.
3.

TRUST IN OCCUPATIONS In terms of the community, who do you trust in terms of occupation?

Rank the following twenty occupations according to the trust you place in them. If you're in a hurry, rank your first five choices and your last five choices.:

auto repairpersons	newspaper columnists
business executives	physicians
clergy	plumbers
college professors	politicians
dentists	psychologists
high school teachers	psychiatrists
judges	TV news reporters
labor union officials	TV repairpersons
law enforcement officers	U.S. Army generals
lawyers	used car salespersons

(Turn to the next page and see how your rankings compare with others).

A team of psychologists from the University of Connecticut surveyed 400 people and found their choices to be as follows:

1. physicians
2. clergy
3. dentists
4. judges
5. psychologists
6. college professors
7. psychiatrists
8. high school teachers
9. lawyers
10. law enforcement officials
11. TV news reporters
12. plumbers
13. business executives
14. U.S. Army generals
15. TV repairpersons
16. newspaper columnists
17. auto repairpersons
18. labor union officials
19. politicians
20. used car salespersons

Why don't you do a survey of your own and find out how trustworthy people think nurses are?

Posttest

1. State a working definition of trust.
   Trust is:

2. Evidence shows that those who trust have which of the following qualities?

   A. comfortable with an increased awareness of self, goals, and motivation
   B. able to share self-awareness with appropriate people
   C. accept others who deviate from their own ways of thinking, feeling, and acting without feeling an intense need to change them
   D. accept new experiences cautiously
   E. demonstrate a consistency between words and actions that lasts over a period of time
   F. unable to delay gratification

3. State three elements of communication that make trust possible.

   A. B. C.

4. Describe two ways to determine if self-disclosure is appropriate in a relationship.

   A.

   B.

5. State the term most commonly confused with trust:

6. Describe the two most common issues related to trust in the nurse-client relationship.

   A.

   B.

7. List the three questions we deal with when we enter a new group.

   A.

   B.

   C.

8. State the two major facets of risk in a group.

   A.

   B.

Posttest Answers

1. The definition must include *to rely upon* or similar meaning.
2. A, B, C, E
3. A. *consistent; congruent; clear*
4. A. Is it reciprocal?
   B. Is the responsibility for the relationship and its depth shared?
5. to tolerate
6. A. The client expects the nurse to tell the truth.
   B. The client asks the nurse to keep secrets.
7. A. Who is involved in this group?
   B. Who has the power?
   C. How close can we get?
8. A. risking to expose oneself
   B. risking to expose another

REFERENCES

1. Carlson, Carolyn E., ed. "Trust in the Nurse-Patient Relationship" *Behavioral Concepts and Nursing Interventions* (Philadelphia: J. B. Lippincott Company, 1970).

2. Egan, Gerard, ed. "One Small-Group Leader's Paradoxical Problems of Becoming a Member of His Own Group," *Encounter Groups: Basic Readings* (Belmont, California: Brooks/Cole Publishing Company, 1971), pp. 144-142.

3. Haley, Jay. *Strategies of Psychotherapy* (New York: Grune and Stratton, 1963), pp. 1-19.

4. Human Development Institute. *Relationship Improvement Program* (Atlanta: HDI, 1967), p. 4.

5. Lederer, William J., and Don D. Jackson. *The Mirages of Marriage* (New York: W. W. Norton and Company, Inc., 1968), pp. 106-113.

6. Lewis, Garland D. *Nurse-Patient Communication* (Dubuque, Iowa: Wm. C. Brown Company, 1973), pp. 67-70.

7. Luft, Joseph. *Of Human Interaction* (Palo Alto, California: National Press Books, 1969), pp. 127-133.

8. Poland, Ronal G. *Human Experience* (Saint Louis: The C. V. Mosby Co., 1974), pp. 16-17.

Support

DIRECTIONS

1. Complete the pretest. If you answer all the questions correctly, you may choose to complete the unit on support for added enrichment and knowledge.

2. After the pretest, complete the activities as directed. The activities and exercises should be completed in the order presented.

3. In order to complete the unit, you will need a pencil and pen. No other materials are needed.

4. A posttest will be given at the end of the unit. Successful completion of this test is necessary for you to have met the objectives.

OBJECTIVES

Upon completion of this unit on support, the learner will be able to:

1. Define support.
2. List at least ten words, ideas, or synonyms associated with support.
3. Describe the importance of support in nursing practice.
4. Describe the concept *interpersonal warmth.*
5. List at least three verbal and three nonverbal supportive behaviors that are commonly manifested.
6. Differentiate antecedent support and consequent support.

7. Identify five forms of antecedent support.
8. Identify four forms of consequent support.
9. Identify five kinds of failure to provide support.
10. Identify four possible problems in receiving support.
11. Formulate a plan for providing support to a nursing client.
12. Describe the concept *support system.*

Pretest

True (T) or False (F)

_____ 1. Support means to uphold by aid, encouragement, or countenance.

_____ 2. Respect, evaluation, and acceptance are congruent with the concept of support.

_____ 3. Clients experiencing minor illness or injury usually require little support.

_____ 4. It is important that health team members be supportive of each other.

_____ 5. The need for interpersonal warmth decreases with age.

_____ 6. Verbal supportive behavior is much more important than nonverbal.

_____ 7. Listening, smiling, and touching are usually supportive in nature.

_____ 8. Antecedent support is that given any time before successful completion of a task or activity.

_____ 9. Reinforcement is synonymous with consequent support.

_____ 10. "Unconditional positive regard" is a form of antecedent support.

_____ 11. Approval is essential to effectively give support.

____ 12. It is possible to provide support even if trust is absent.

____ 13. Recognition and response should occur together for effective support.

____ 14. Immediate reinforcement is more supportive than delayed response.

____ 15. Not all empathy is accurate and effective as support.

____ 16. Although it sounds trite, stating, "I know how you feel," is usually very supportive.

____ 17. A dependency conflict often blocks an individual from receiving support.

____ 18. Being supportive to another person involves recognizing his or her strengths.

____ 19. As long as the objective is a positive health behavior, it is supportive to manipulate an individual.

____ 20. Each person has a unique support system and individual ways of getting and giving support.

Pretest Answers

1. True	2. False	3. False	4. True	5. False	6. False
7. True	8. False	9. True	10. True	11. False	12. False
13. True	14. True	15. True	16. False	17. True	
18. True	19. False	20. True			

INTRODUCTION

Men resemble the gods in nothing so much as in doing good to their fellow creatures.

Cicero

According to a dictionary, *support* means: "to bear; to sustain; to uphold by aid, encouragement, or countenance; to keep from fainting, sinking, failing or declining." Utilizing this definition as a frame of reference, think about the word *support*. Write, in the space below, fifteen words that come quickly to mind when you think of psychological support. Do not attempt to find any sense of order in the words.

1.	6.	11.
2.	7.	12.
3.	8.	13.
4.	9.	14.
5.	10.	15.

Many responses are possible. Psychological support readily suggests:

encouragement, respect
acceptance, psychological safety
regard, nonevaluative
reinforcement, warmth
empathy, understanding
concern, compassion
trust, recognition
responsiveness, sympathy
comfort
nonjudgmental
perhaps, agape!, or even, love

As a nurse, you are frequently called upon to give support to clients. Health problems, even minor ones, can disrupt an individual's life style, family relationships, and work productivity. Consequently, he or she will need assistance in coping with the disruption; this assistance should be an integral part of his or her plan of care. Nursing is not restricted to performing activities or doing procedures. Much needed support might be provided by effective listening, supplying information and answering questions, pleasant conversation, and, very important, allowing and encouraging the client to maintain his or her independence to whatever degree is possible.

Important too is that as you work with colleagues, other health team members, and other individuals, you will find that your support is required by all of them, most of them, or some of them, to a degree. To perform your daily work well, and to communicate effectively, you will need to develop your abilities to their fullest potential so that your capacity to give support is not depleted.

In relation to the above, O'Brien has formulated some questions for reflection (1974, pp. 53-54).

1. Can you give support by words but not by your actions?

2. Do you constantly give encouragement so that others are dependent on you?

3. Are you able to give support to another only to the degree that it is requested?

4. Will you assist others so that they can retain their dignity and composure?

5. Will you be hopeful and optimistic to others so that they can feel your support?

6. Do you see another in distress and not offer support because you cannot extend yourself?

7. Do you shield yourself from pain while another is experiencing grief or sorrow?

8. Can you not support others because you have not been encouraged?

9. Do you realize that our society does not place a *value* on encouraging others but, rather, that emphasis is given to competing with them?

Unfortunately, success at any cost is the formula followed by many in our country. We have lost the art of being human with one another and of being comfortable with other people who are not familiar to us (O'Brien, 1974, p. 54).

This module, then, is designed to help you begin to deal with the above questions and issues. The content is based, to a great extent, on Egan's excellent conceptual framework; and although not required for this module, you are strongly encouraged to study his writing.

NEED FOR SUPPORT Recognizing the universal need for *interpersonal warmth* is important to understanding the concept of support. A degree of warmth in interpersonal relationships is essential for psychological growth and development. This need begins at birth; and although it might undergo transformations throughout the maturational process, it is still a strongly felt need during old age. Therefore, since the nurse-client relationship is obviously interpersonal, a climate of support and psychological safety must exist. What would happen if this climate were not present?

Consider these questions. Space is provided for you to give a brief response.

1. From what people in my life have I felt the most support?

2. What was it they did that was supportive?

3. How did they give support? Physically? Emotionally? Intellectually? Spiritually?

4. What feelings did I have as I was receiving support?

5. To what people in my life have I provided the most support?

6. What feelings did I have as I was giving support?

7. How did I handle these feelings?

8. What specific behaviors can I identify as supportive behaviors? List five verbal and five nonverbal behaviors that would be supportive. Remember that "behaviors" must be observable and measurable. Possible responses appear following yours.

Verbal	Nonverbal
1.	1.
2.	2.
3.	3.
4.	4.
5.	5.

Verbal	Nonverbal
1. I like you.	1. smiling
2. You are a nice person.	2. active listening
3. I will help you.	3. touch of hand
4. I'm glad I know you.	4. arm around shoulder
5. You can handle it.	5. looking at speaker
6. Any sincere compliment.	6. nodding of head
7. I will listen to you.	7. leaning toward speaker
8. I need your feedback.	8. hugging (not a "bear" hug)
9. I need your help.	9. silence—sometimes
10. I respect your opinion.	10. stroking head, as when comforting

Did your list include others?

Whether verbal or nonverbal, there are basically two kinds of support: antecedent and consequent. Direct or indirect encouragement to engage in behavior or a relationship is *antecedent* support; that is, it comes before behavior and is directed toward eliciting it. For example, a nurse might approach a client stating, "Hello, my name is Jane Brown." This simple act supports and encourages clients to introduce themselves, thereby beginning a relationship. On the other hand, reinforcement given for action, interaction, or for actually engaging in behavior, is *consequent* support. Encouragement and comfort given to a woman in labor, for example, "I know it's difficult for you, but you're doing a fine job of following instructions," falls into this category. You can surely think of other illustrations, but let us explore some forms of each type of support.

ANTECEDENT SUPPORT *Acceptance*, sometimes called "unconditional positive regard," is a form of antecedent support. Accepting a client for who he or she is, what he or she is, or simply because he or she *is*, sounds deceptively easy; but in reality, this attitude is often difficult to convey. Each of us, including you, has biases and prejudices that block the basic acceptance of certain people. List traits, characteristics, or behaviors that interfere with your giving "unconditional positive regard."

1.
2.
3.
4.
5.
6.
7.
8.
9.
10.

If you had difficulty responding, you might need to do some "soul searching" or introspection to develop more self-awareness. Remember, it is human and inevitable that, even as an intelligent adult, you will have prejudices. The trick is to be aware of them and to learn how to deal with them so that they do not severely hinder your ability to give support and adequate health care.

In relation to the above, it is important to differentiate *acceptance* and *approval*. The latter is not necessarily required for the former. Acceptance indicates, "I accept you, where you are, but I might not approve of your behavior or what you are doing." List persons or clients whom you believe you could accept, but whose actions or activities you could not condone.

1.
2.
3.
4.
5.
6.
7.
8.
9.
10.

Compare this list with the previous one. There will likely be similarities *and* differences. What does this mean concerning your providing acceptance, approval, and support to all clients needing your nursing services?

Expressing a sense of solidarity in the "human condition" is a significant form of antecedent support. Harry Stack Sullivan once said, "We are all much more alike than we are dissimilar." What does this mean to you? Do you believe it to be true? List those activities, problems, or needs of living that you see as being experienced by most or all "mere humans."

1.	6.
2.	7.
3.	8.
4.	9.
5.	10.

The following are possible responses. If you had difficulty thinking of responses, take a few minutes and consider each of the given responses and how it is part of the "human condition."

The most obvious responses would be *birth* and *death*. Others might be:

physiological activities—breathing,
eating,
sleeping, and so on

emotions and feeling—anger,
sadness,
joy,
elation,
depression, and so on

activities—work,
play,
hobbies, and so on

needs—nourishment, shelter, clothing, recreation,
and don't forget, *interpersonal warmth*

Another form of antecedent support is *availability*. This is important on both an individual and collective basis, for how can clients avail themselves of health services, and strive to high-level wellness, if nurses and health care are not accessible and readily available? What implications can you see regarding the planning and delivery of nursing and health care services? On a more individual level, can you recall situations where nonavailability interfered with, or blocked, a client getting the support he or she needed and deserved? Although these questions are somewhat rhetorical, you will be dealing with them for the rest of your nursing career. I wish you luck.

Authenticity, or *congruence*, is a form of antecedent support, and is essential for a working relationship between nurse and client. Role-playing, insincerity, and "unreal" behavior will inhibit communication and support almost immediately. An illustration of incongruence frequently encountered is perceived differences in verbal and nonverbal behavior. How do you react to a friend telling you, "I am too listening!" when he or she is turned away and looking intently at another person? Do you feel supported? What other examples of incongruence or nonauthenticity have you encountered as a nurse or in your personal experience? Write a brief description of one. Identify the conflicting "messages" conveyed. How did the receiver react or respond?

Incongruence:

Messages (at least two):

1.

2.

3.

4.

Response:

The last form of antecedent support to be identified is *trust formation*. Trust is very important, since without it, it is impossible to give and receive support. Also, you will need to work actively toward creating a climate of trust with your client, because the trust-mistrust conflict is almost an inherent part of the human condition. Recall the module on trust. Whom do you trust? What symptoms of distrust do you experience? Have you ever undergone misplaced trust or confidence? What was your reaction? A feeling of betrayal? Shame? Embarrassment? Have you encountered clients who find it difficult to trust you? Why should your clients trust you? What can you do to foster trust and confidence in your providing nursing care and services? Are you overwhelmed by all these questions? Sorry. Take a moment to relax before continuing.

CONSEQUENT SUPPORT It has been stated that consequent support is synonymous with reinforcement. Therefore, the principles of good reinforcement technique would apply to consequent support. One of these principles is that *recognition and appropriate response* should occur together; ideally they will merge into a single act. It is not enough for the nurse to simply recognize a client's behavior. An appropriate response is needed for the reinforcement to be supportive. For example, a nurse telling a client, "You've learned to walk with crutches now," might add for support, "You execute crutch walking very well," or, "Now that you can walk with crutches, you won't have to wait for someone to bring you things." Also, "appropriate" response implies reinforcing in proportion to the value of the behavior. It would be nonsupportive for the nurse to tell a client, "Now that you can walk with crutches, you can completely resume your normal functioning." Why would this be untrue, and therefore, unsupportive?

Important too is the *immediacy of reinforcement.* How supportive would it be if a nurse told a client, "Yesterday, when you did your colostomy care for the first time, you did a fine job"? Would it not have been better to state, at that time, "Considering this is the first time to do this, you're doing a fine job of learning to do your colostomy care"?

Along with immediacy, *accurate empathy* is essential for support. This refers to the ability of the nurse to understand, accurately and sensitively, experiences and feelings and their meaning to the client. Consider the following responses:

> "Mr. Jones, you shouldn't find your colostomy care distasteful. After all, expelling feces is a natural body process."

or

> "Mr. Jones, I can understand your finding your colostomy care distasteful. Tell me more about how you feel about doing it."

Which is the more supportive? Which reflects more an accurate empathy on the part of the nurse? You will see later in the module how empathy can be distorted or misused. For now, consider for a moment what empathy means, and how it differs from sympathy. Although somewhat supportive, sympathy too often is disguised pity, and a client will seldom find pity supportive or encouraging.

Lastly regarding consequent support, clients need and deserve *individual reinforcement* rather than as one of a group. For instance, consider a nurse telling a diabetic client who is anxious about learning to administer his or her own insulin, "Don't worry. Anyone can learn to give his or her own injections." Write a more supportive statement.

If you were doing health teaching to a group of expectant mothers, and one woman stated, "I understand the natural childbirth method, and I want to use it, but I'm afraid I won't be able to stand the pain," how would you answer, using individual reinforcement? Write your response.

Write a response that would neglect the client's individuality.

FAILURES IN SUPPORT A nurse might fail to support clients in a variety of ways. One of these is the *cliche* or *ritualistic support.* A good example of this is the socially acceptable cliche, attempting to express support, "I know how you feel." Since no one can truly "know" how another feels, this socialized statement is not supportive. At its worst, using "I know how you feel" is followed by "because I . . ." This serves to divert attention from the supportee's situation, and denies the validity of his or her own feelings and experience.

Another failure is *cheap empathy.* This is distorted and misused empathy, often conveying pity, and seems to be directed toward fulfilling the needs of the one giving support rather than the one in need. Persons using this failure resemble "professional mourners," never missing a chance to give support, especially to one suffering. It might also manifest itself as oversupport or "mush." If you have ever encountered a well-meaning, but glibly gushed, "I understand. You poor thing," you will recognize this inept attempt to be supportive. Who needs it?!

Egan also describes the *St. Sebastian Syndrome,* named after the

Christian martyr who was killed, it is reported, by being shot full of arrows. This occurs when support would be an appropriate response, but the one attempting it does not know how to go about it. Therefore, he or she responds with a barrage of questions, for example, "How do you feel?" "How are things now?" "How long has it been going on?" If this continues for long, the one in need of support loses awareness of whatever feelings needed supporting. This does not mean that an occasional question cannot be insightful and supportive, but it must be appropriate, nonritualistic, sincere, and not one of Twenty Questions thrown at someone needing support.

Persons who do *"Red Crossing"* or *rescuing* cannot tolerate seeing another in any kind of pain or discomfort, physical or emotional, even if it might be beneficial to the individual. They quickly try to aid the sufferer by rationalizing away the discomfort or taking immediate measure to alleviate it. Nurses frequently misuse pain relievers, tranquilizers, or sleep medication in an effort to "erase" clients' complaints or distress. Needless to say, the red crosser seldom offers real support, but only palliative softeners.

Silence, if it is protracted or overused, can fail to be supportive. In these cases, it usually serves to precipitate anxiety and suppression of feelings. How long a silence can you tolerate when talking with someone? How might you interpret silence if you wanted a supportive reaction or response?

Problems in Receiving Support

Since support is so important to nursing process and practice, a brief discussion of problems in receiving support will be presented. Keep in mind that these problems may be exhibited by yourself, your clients or other members of the health team. If problems rear their ugly heads, you will need to do some analysis and incorporate "solutions" into your plan of care or action.

An individual may be experiencing a *dependency-independency conflict* with which he or she has been struggling. This will surely detract from his or her ability to receive support. Another person difficult to support is the one who thrives on support and encouragement. His or her exaggerated need may drive the person to groveling or obsequious behavior to get your approval. The need is valid, but your patience will be tried in attempting to meet the need appropriately.

Lack of trust, pervasive or sparse, will inhibit an individual's receiving support. The only solution is to work at establishing trust—even a small amount is better than none. Also, you will likely encounter people who, for whatever reason, have a persistent need to maintain social pleasantness in their relationships. They are easily threatened by more than superficial interactions, and will block any attempt to provide support.

There are no easy solutions to these problems. Other than recognizing and being aware of their existence, you may have little success dealing with them. When this happens, you will have to accept your status as "human." This means simply that you will not succeed at everything you attempt to do. Is occasional failure okay with you? Can you give support and encouragement to yourself? "Be not too hard, for life is short, and little is given to man." (Source unknown)

Now that you have learned everything you have always wanted to know about support—but were afraid to ask?—you may well ask, "How can I utilize all this in nursing?" Good question! One of the most effective ways to provide support is by reinforcing another person's strengths. Being supportive can be defined as communicating to another person that you recognize his or her strengths and believe the person has the capabilities of handling productively whatever situation he or she faces.

Everyone builds upon his or her strengths. As individuals become more aware of their strengths, and more able to demonstrate their strengths, they will gain the self-confidence needed to overcome stress and disruptions such as those caused by illness and/or health problems. Reinforcement is helpful in providing support and encouraging constructive behavior by giving strengthening feedback immediately after the person has engaged in a behavior that: (1) demonstrates one of these strengths; or (2) indicates an attempt to overcome a barrier to the expression of his or her strengths. The following exercise will provide practice in doing this (Johnson, 1972), pp. 181-183).

1. Think of a client with whom you are working, or have worked with, (a) whose problem-solving skills you could help improve; (b) who lacks the self-confidence to utilize his or her skills, or (c) to whom you would like to express more support. This "client" may be a friend, lover, family member, or an individual from your clinical experience. In the space below, describe the person's basic strengths.

2. What are the barriers that keep this person from expressing or utilizing his or her strengths? Examples of barriers are a lack of self-confidence, fear of rejection, fear that people will think he or she is foolish, wanting to be overly nice, or lack of self-acceptance. You will likely be able to identify others. The barriers for this person are:

3. What are the possible strengthening consequences you could provide for this person? Examples of strengthening consequences are the expression of warmth, acceptance, encouragement, understanding, self-disclosure about your positive reactions to his or her behavior, and others that have been discussed in this module. The strengthening consequences that I could provide for this person are:

4. Reviewing what you have listed in Steps 1, 2, and 3, write at least two behavioral objectives for your interactions with the person for the following week. The objectives should include a statement of countable behavior on the part of the person, directionality of change in the countable behavior, and a description of countable behavior by you to provide a strengthening consequence. Such a behavioral objective might be, "increase the number of times John initiates a conversation by expressing warmth towards him immediately after he does so in my presence." My objectives are:

5. Review your objectives. It is important that they not be attempts to manipulate the other person, but rather expressions of support for behaviors you believe will facilitate the person's expression of his or her strengths or the elimination of barriers to the demonstration of his or her strengths. Your objectives should reflect a sincere attempt to be supportive, not an attempt to remake the other person. On the basis of your review, rewrite any objectives that may seem more manipulative than supportive.

6. During the next week, keep a "record sheet" as outlined below. At the end of the week, review the sheet to explore the relationship between the number of strengthening consequences you engaged in and the number of times the other person engaged in behaviors that demonstrated his or her strengths or attempts to overcome barriers to utilizing these strengths.

Record Sheet

	Number of times other person engaged in behavior to be increased	Number of times I engaged in a strengthening consequence
Day One		
Day Two		
Day Three		
Day Four		
Day Five		
Day Six		
Day Seven		

Brief mention will be made of the concept of *support system.* Utilizing a dictionary definition of *system* (an arrangement of things so related as to form a unity or whole) plus the definition of *support* (recall from beginning of module), you can see that support system refers to the organized way in which an individual gets the encouragement and interpersonal warmth he or she needs. This includes the person's activities (work, play, recreation, and so on) and the significant others with whom he or she interacts regularly (parents, siblings, spouse, children, friends, lovers, and so on). Outline your support system by listing the activities and people in it, in order of most to least supportive.

Activities

1.
2.
3.
4.
5.
6.

People

1.
2.
3.
4.
5.
6.
7.
8.
9.
10.

Keep in mind that this support system reflects who, what, and where you are right now. It probably has changed from five years ago, and will undergo further revision in your future. Also, you should recognize that it is *your* support system, and it may be similar, but not identical to anyone else's. You will need to remember this in your nursing practice. Each client (and others with whom you work) will have his or her own unique support system and individual ways of getting and giving support. In your clinical experience, make an effort to identify your clients' support systems, and incorporate them into your nursing care plans.

Lastly, give attention to O'Brien's thoughtful words (1974, p. 54):

> Let us endeavor, to whatever degree is possible, to demonstrate encouragement in our daily activities. It can be in the form of a word, a smile, a letter, a call, a touch, a thank you, a gentle manner, a courteous greeting, a listening ear, your presence while another is experiencing some difficulty, or your performing activities that the other person would do if he had the strength, ability, or emotional control. All of us can, in our own ways and in our own areas, make the world a nicer place in which to live, for ourselves and others.

You have completed this module. Thank you for your attention and participation. Complete the posttest and check your answers. And be good to yourself—you deserve it.

Posttest

Circle the correct answer.

1. Which of the following is *not* a definition of support?

   A. to uphold by aid, encouragement, or countenance

   B. communicating to another person that you recognize his or her strengths

   C. to manage or control negative behavior

   D. to keep from sinking, failing, or declining

2. Which ones of the following are congruent with the concept of support?

   A. encouragement

   B. respect

   C. evaluation

   D. dependency

   E. indifference

   F. psychological safety

   G. regard

   H. judgment

   I. manipulation

   J. reinforcement

3. Which of the following is *not* true of interpersonal warmth?

   A. It indicates a universal need.

   B. The need begins at birth and ends only at death.

   C. It is essential for growth and development.

   D It is of minor importance in a professional, nurse-client relationship.

4. Which of the following would *not* be considered supportive?

A. I like you.
B. I respect your opinion.
C. You must do as I say.
D. You can do it yourself.
E. Your hair looks nice today.
F. I know what's best for you.

1. C, D, E
2. D, E, F
3. C, F
4. none of the above

5. Which of the following usually would be supportive?

A. smiling
B. active listening
C. a "bear" hug
D. leaning toward speaker
E. frowning
F. stroking leg

1. A, C, D
2. A, B, D
3. A, B, D, F
4. B, C, D, F

6. Which of the following is *not* a form of antecedent support?

A. acceptance
B. unconditional approval
C. availability
D. congruence
E. trust formation

7. Which of the following is *not* a form of consequent support?

A. recognition and appropriate response
B. immediate reinforcement
C. sharing "human condition"
D. accurate empathy
E. individual reinforcement

8. Match the failure in support (letter) with the appropriate description (number).

    A. ritualistic support

    B. cheap empathy

    C. St. Sebastian syndrome

    D. Red Crossing

    E. silence

1. rescuing with palliative softeners
2. a socially appropriate cliché
3. barrage of insincere questions
4. protracted; precipitates anxiety
5. pity, oversupport, or "mush"

9. Match the problem in receiving support (letter) with the appropriate symptom (number).

    A. dependency conflict

    B. thriving on encouragement

    C. lack of trust

    D. maintaining social pleasantness

1. obsequious behavior
2. superficial interaction
3. defensive reaction
4. suspicious attitude

10. In reinforcing another person's strengths, which of the following is *most* supportive? Communicating that you recognize his or her strengths and:

    A. will help the person with his or her weaknesses.

    B. believe that he or she can handle any situation appropriately.

    C. will help the person compensate for his or her weaknesses.

    d. do not see his or her weaknesses.

11. Which of the following is *not* true of the concept *support system*?

    A. It is fixed by adulthood, and seldom changes after that.

    B. It is the organized way in which one gets encouragement and warmth.

    C. Support systems are unique for each individual.

    D. It includes a person's activities and significant others.

12. All of the following describe the importance of support in your nursing practice except:

    A. Anyone experiencing a health problem is in need of support.

    B. To one degree or another, other health team members will require your support.

    C. At times, you will need to give support and encouragement to yourself.

    D. It is most effective to formulate supportive measures separate from nursing care plan.

Posttest Answers

1. C 2. A, B, F, G, J 3. D 4. 3 5. 2 6. B 7. C
8. A. 2, B. 5; C. 3, D. 1, E. 4 9. A. 3, B. 1, C. 4, D. 2 10. B
11. A 12. D

REFERENCES

1. Egan, Gerard. *Encounter: Group Processes for Interpersonal Growth* (Belmont, California: Brooks/Cole Publishing Co., 1970), pp. 260-286.

2. Johnson, David W. *Reaching Out* (Englewood Cliffs, New Jersey: Prentice-Hall, Inc., 1972), pp. 141-157, 171-187.

3. O'Brien, Maureen J. *Communications and Relationships in Nursing* (St. Louis: C. V. Mosby Co., 1974), pp. 53-55, 62-63, 117-119.

Listening

DIRECTIONS

1. Complete the pretest. If you answer all the questions correctly, you may choose to complete the unit on listening for added enrichment and knowledge.

2. After the pretest, complete the activities as directed. The activities and exercises should be completed in the order presented.

3. In order to complete the unit, you will need a pencil or pen. No other materials are needed.

4. A posttest will be given at the end of the unit. Successful completion of this test is necessary for you to have met the unit objectives.

OBJECTIVES

Upon completion of this unit on listening, the learner will be able to:

1. Define listening.

2. Name the four steps of the process of effective listening.

3. List the four major components of the concept *Total Listening.*

4. List and give examples of three levels of listening.

5. Identify and differentiate three major obstacles to effective listening.

6. Explain the importance of effective listening in nursing practice.

7. List six specific benefits of effective listening.

8. Identify four guidelines for effective listening.

Pretest

True (T) or False (F)

1. "Listening" and "hearing" are not necessarily the same thing.

2. Listening is a passive process whereby a person gives his or her attention to another so that he or she can hear what is being said.

3. Coding, inferring, and interpretation are important steps in the listening process.

4. Listening includes the act of responding to total messages.

5. Total Listening requires the listener to be selective, active, and socially intelligent.

6. Detecting what is not said (listening with "Third Ear") is important to Total Listening.

7. For effective listening, the listener must remain totally silent.

8. Content and feelings are understood on two different levels of listening.

9. "I feel sad today," indicates a set or pattern in the speaker's reaction to situations.

10. It is usually effective for a listener to formulate a response while a person is speaking.

11. It is impossible to listen effectively if a person is telling you something you do *not* want to hear.

12. External preoccupation and anxiety are common barriers to listening.

13. Past experience can cause a listener to distort a speaker's message.

14. It is often useful for a listener to "round off" what he or she hears, thereby dividing the content into clear-cut messages.

15. Listeners often modify messages so that they conform to an expected meaning.

16. "Just listening" usually provides little support to the speaker.

17. Effective listening is a valuable tool in the planning of nursing care.

18. Listening is most important in a psychiatric setting where a "therapeutic" nurse-client relationship is the goal.

19. It is essential to establish contact and use no gestures when listening.

20. Paraphrasing, clarifying, and perception checking are useful skills for effective listening.

Pretest Answers

1. True	2. False	3. True	4. True	5. False	6. True
7. False	8. True	9. False	10. False	11. False	12. True
13. True	14. False	15. True	16. False	17. True	
18. False	19. False	20. True			

INTRODUCTION

Were we as eloquent as angels,
yet should we please some men
and some women much more by
listening than by talking. *COLTON*

A dictionary defines listening as making a conscious effort to hear; attending closely so as to hear. To expound on this definition, here are a few other explanations and descriptions by selected writers.

> At first glance the term *listening* implies a passive act of taking in the content of the helpee's communication, but actually it involves a very active process of responding to total messages. It includes not only listening with the ears to his words and with the eyes to his body language, but a total kind of perceptiveness which is best described by Reik's (1948) term "listening with the third ear" . . . . When the helper can answer in considerable detail the question, 'What is going on in this person right now and in his life space?" He is listening with all his perceptual capacities. Listening skills are basic to all interviewing whether the purpose be for gaining information, conducting structured depth interviews, or open informal helping (Brammer, 1973, pp. 81-82).

> For our purposes, listening means becoming aware of all the cues that the other emits, and this implies an openness to the totality of the communication of the other (Egan, 1970, p. 248).

> It seems pertinent to make the distinction between hearing and listening . . . "To hear" means specifically to become aware of sounds. It is essentially a passive thing, occurring automatically when sound waves stimulate the auditory nerves. "To listen" requires one to make an active, conscious effort to attend closely to the auditory stimuli. The distinction between the two words lies in "the conscious effort" required for listening, which makes it more active than just hearing a sound (Lewis, 1973, p. 37).

> Thus the ear serves a double function in communication: physiologically for the reception of sound, and psychologically for the perception of attitudes associated with words. (Lewis, 1973, p. 36).

> Listening is an art or skill whereby a person consciously and voluntarily gives his attention to another so that he can hear what is being said. Listening is not a passive process. Rather, it requires your utmost concentration and effort. To be effective in the process of communication, you must accept the responsibility both to speak well and to listen attentively when another speaks (O'Brien, 1974, p. 33).

EFFECTIVE LISTENING

Based on the definitions, explanations and descriptions given in the introduction, a process of *effective* listening can be formulated. Put the steps described below in their logical sequence.

a. inferring and interpreting—organizing all the transmitted cues into a message that has meaning in the speaker's framework

b. perceiving and hearing—receiving sensory stimuli and transmitting them to cognitive centers in the brain

c. responding—conveying to the speaker that he or she is being listened to, and that the messages are understood

d. active coding—translating sensory input into rational signs and symbols that make sense for the listener

1.

2.

3.

4.

ANSWERS

1. b 2. d 3. a 4. c

If your responses were incorrect, review the steps to see the correct order.

The concept of listening can be expanded, for further clarification, to what Egan calls *Total Listening* (Egan, 1970, pp. 248-252). This view of listening seems most complete, but you may hear *active* or *effective* used to modify the word *listening*, meaning pretty much the same thing. List three other adjectives that would describe, and strengthen the activity of, listening.

1.

2.

3.

Possible responses are below.

"Good" listening can be said to be:

Complete

Thorough

Holistic

Responsive

Efficient

Cogent

Functional, Operative, Receptive

Whatever your responses, for now consider Total Listening. Total Listening is nonselective (verbal *and* nonverbal messages are received), active (not passive), and socially intelligent (feeling for people and involving oneself creatively and responsibly with them) (Egan, 1970, pp. 249-252). It includes O'Brien's readiness to engage and receptivity to new ideas, along with the listener detecting what is not said (O'Brien, 1974, pp. 36-38). Also, creative and efficacious use of silence is required for listening to be effective (Lewis, 1973, pp. 40-44). What might happen to the speaker if silence is misused or overused? The answer is simple—he would very likely become anxious and stop talking, thereby blocking communication.

As a review exercise, list four major components of Total Listening. Sort the above words and ideas into four categories.

1.

2.

3.

4.

ANSWERS

1. *nonselectivity,* including listening with "third ear"
2. *social intelligence,* including readiness and receptivity to new ideas
3. *active engagement* in the communication process
4. *silence* used appropriately and productively

If your responses are not exactly as above, you may want to review the information on Total Listening. However, you are allowed (even encouraged) to formulate your own categories as long as they make sense to you. The posttest, though, will cover the above components.

Consider the following conversation:

You: And that's happened a number of times. I'm about to move away from home.

I: You are considering moving.

You: Well, I'm close to it. I just don't want to be dominated all the time.

I: It bugs you to be told what to do.

You: Yes, I want them to stop telling me what to do, and I'm going to tell them that. It's always like that. People think I have no feelings, and they can walk all over me.

I: It happens other places too, but this time you're going to tell them to stop doing it.

You: I sure will.

In the conversation, my responses have attempted to encourage you to go on, and come to your own conclusion. This listening was done on three different levels.

1. I fed back *content*—"You are considering moving."

2. A richer kind of listening occurred when I also picked up your *feeling*—"It bugs you . . ."

3. I got to an even more basic level when I listened for a *set* or *pattern*—"It happens other places too . . ." A "set" indicates a readiness to respond in a certain way to situations, and is based on a pervasive feeling about him or herself that a person carries around, for example, "No one cares what I think," or "I always do it wrong." This feeling determines, to a great extent, how somebody will react in particular situations, and if a listener can reach this level, the contact becomes most meaningful.

On all three levels, it is important to give feedback that indicates acceptance of what is said as being true for the speaker. If a speaker's statements are rephrased in a challenging way, they will probably cause him or her to become defensive and stop the flow of thought. Example:

I: Do you *really* believe they dominate you?

You: Of course they do! Why, yesterday even . . .
and your energy goes into defending and proving your statement.

Read the following statements, and write three responses that indicate listening on each of the levels.

I think I'll withdraw from school. I'm worried as hell that I didn't pass the last test. I'm not surprised though; I always do lousy on exams.

1. Content:

2. Feeling:

3. Set or Pattern:

A good question now is—what stops, or gets in the way of, listening effectively? You can likely formulate some answers yourself. As food for thought, consider the following "barriers to hearing" set forth by O'Brien (1974, pp. 33–34).

You have difficulty hearing the words of another when

—the person's views are different from yours

—the person's culture, education, or work experience deviates from yours

—it is not easy to follow the thoughts expressed because the vocabulary is not known to you

—the person speaks with a dialect or accent

—the attire or appearance of the speaker is extreme in some way

—you have heard the discourse before by the speaker or someone else

—the thoughts or feelings being expressed shock you or cause you to feel anxious

—you realize you are out of your depth in trying to converse with another

—the person is telling you something you *do not* want to hear

—the environment is noisy, or frequent interruptions occur

—you are experiencing stress or discomfort to any degree (physical, emotional, social)

—the words of the speaker belie his or her actions or true feelings

—your emotions influence your rational approach to the discourse

—you will have to admit an error

—you realize an apology from you should be forthcoming

—the values you support are under attack

—you are self-centered and hear only your own voice

—the news or outcome of a situation is not good

—the needs of another will demand a commitment or involvement by you

—a physical condition develops and the sense of hearing is impaired or lost permanently

—you decide you dislike the person, with insufficient information or evidence

This list may have seemed "long-winded." Well, it was. Perhaps easier to understand and remember are the "obstacles to effective listening" outlined by Egan (1970, pp. 252–258). His three major categories are:

1. *Alienation from Communication.* This includes preoccupation with external events, self-consciousness (self-preoccupation), and interaction-consciousness (being so worried about how the interaction is progressing that ability to follow conversation is constricted).

2. *Message Anxiety.* This blocks listening when the content of a message is anxiety-arousing for the speaker and/or the listener. It can become cyclic if the speaker conveys anxious feeling to the listener, who picks up the feeling and, not being in touch with it or dealing with it, reconveys the feeling back to the speaker.

3. *Human Error in the Communication Process.* This category covers sources of systematic error in human interaction which inhibit effective communication. Developed by D.T. Campbell (1958), they include:

   a. speaker's remarks are too long

   b. middle of the message is least well retained

   c. listener tends to "round off" what he or she hears

   d. imperfectly transmitted messages are distorted in the direction of important past messages

   e. a new message is modified so that it becomes more like previous messages

   f. message is modified so it is in better agreement with listener's own opinions and attitudes

   g. message is modified to conform to the meaning expected by the listener

h. message is distorted in direction of evaluative coding; that is, black-or-white listening; for example, good vs. bad, beautiful vs. ugly, and so on

i. message is distorted or "filtered" in response to group pressure

Note: You probably will not remember each of these, but they provide helpful principles for improving the purpose of speaking and the process of listening.

To review these obstacles, refer back to O'Brien's list of "barriers," and determine whether each can be classified as (1) alienation from communication, (2) message anxiety, or (3) human error. No answers will be provided, but the exercise will give you a chance to "stretch your mind." Ready. Get set. Stretch!

Why is it important for nurses to be good listeners? If the answer to this question seems obvious, that's okay—it should be obvious to you. The nurse-client relationship is interpersonal, and meaningful interpersonal interaction requires effective listening. More specifically, the following can be derived from active listening:

1. "Just listening" can provide much valuable *support* to clients.
2. Listening is an important *diagnostic* tool, for example, in obtaining nursing history and developing nursing care plans.
3. *Continued observation* utilizes a holistic listening process.
4. Listening provides *"fuel" for effective interaction* between nurse and client.
5. Total listening is essential for establishing and maintaining a *therapeutic relationship.*
6. Not the least of benefits is that by listening, a nurse can *learn*—from clients, from colleagues, from friends, and yes, even from teachers.

Can you formulate additional gains from "good" listening?

The art of listening would be easy if everyone could be clear and direct when they are speaking. However, this is not the case. People in general, and especially clients experiencing illness or health problems, are often inhibited from directness by:

—fear of being rejected

—anxiety about the impact of the words or thoughts on another

—desire to always be accepted

—strong need for approval

—inability to take the risk of stating the thoughts clearly, for then they cannot be retracted

—content of the dialogue that is upsetting to the speaker

—fear of moral judgments being passed

—inability to accept changes that may be required because of the dialogue

—fear that the listener may not view them favorably

—a realization that what is, is not good, but that a confrontation may diminish even the present state

—fear of loss

These factors were formulated by O'Brien (1974, p. 38). They indicate that clients will vary in their ability to discuss what concerns them; thus, they may rely on the nurse to give them assistance.

Learning the skill of effective listening may seem very difficult. It is important though that you recognize that it indeed can be learned. Poor listening habits can be corrected; you can get valuable chances to do this with practice in experiential learning activities and in utilizing what you learn when working with clients. To start you on your way, a few guidelines for listening will be presented as developed by Brammer (1973, pp. 81–87).

1. Attending
    a. Establish contact through looking at the speaker when he talks.
    b. Maintain a natural relaxed posture which indicates your interest.
    c. Use natural gestures which communicate your intended messages.
    d. Use verbal statements which relate to his statements without interruptions, questions, or new topics.

2. Paraphrasing

   a. Listen for the basic message of the speaker.

   b. Restate to the speaker a concise and simple summary of his basic message.

   c. Observe cues or ask for a response from the speaker which confirms or denies the accuracy and helpfulness of the paraphrase for promoting his understanding

3. Clarifying

   a. Admit confusion about speaker's meaning.

   b. Try a restatement or ask for clarification, repetition, or illustration.

4. Perception Checking

   a. Paraphrase what you think you heard.

   b. Ask for confirmation directly from the speaker about the accuracy of your perception of what he said.

   c. Allow the speaker to correct your perception if it was inaccurate.

In the beginning, you may want to use some helpful phrases to preface your feedback, for example, "You feel . . .", "I hear you say . . .", or "Let me see if I understood you . . ." Later on you will become less mechanical, capture the essence of what is said and fit your feedback in, in a way that minimally disrupts the flow of the person to whom you are listening. If your feedback is not accepted by the speaker, do not put energy into proving that you were right or explaining why you thought it was what he or she meant. Instead, ask what the person does mean. To help you develop skill in effective (active, total, and so on) listening, ask your friends to be speakers as you listen. After all, what are friends for? Also, they will undoubtedly learn from the experience too.

You have now completed this module. Complete the posttest, and check your answers. Thank you for your attention and participation. And I wish you—*Good Listening!*

Posttest

Posttest . . .

Circle the correct answer, unless otherwise directed.

1. Which of the following is *not* a definition of listening?

   A. Making a conscious effort to hear; attending closely so as to hear.

   B. An art or skill whereby a person gives his or her attention to another so that he or she can hear what is being said.

   C. A passive act of taking in the content of a speaker's communication when sound waves stimulate the auditory nerves.

   D. Becoming aware of all cues emitted by another and being open to the totality of communication of the other.

2. The process of effective listening includes all of the following except:

   A. perceiving and hearing stimuli

   B. active coding of input

   C. inferring and interpreting cues

   D. evaluating messages

   E. responding verbally and nonverbally

3. All of the following are components of *Total Listening* except:

   A. nonselectivity

   B. social intelligence

   C. active engagement

   D. complete silence

4. Match the appropriate level (number) with the given listening responses (letter).

   A. It made you angry.

   B. It's always this way.

   C. You wrote the person a letter.

   D. You never think you're adequate.

   E. The person's reaction embarrassed you.

   F. She broke your glasses.

      1. content
      2. feeling
      3. set or pattern

5. Which of the following feedback statements does *not* indicate acceptance?

   A. You feel neglected by the person.

   B. They don't actually ignore you, do they?

   C. He didn't tell you he was angry.

   D. She didn't even say goodbye to you.

6. Match the obstacles to listening (number with the given situations (letter).

   A. Watching the patient in the next bed to make sure he or she does not remove his or her IV.

   B. Not being able to recall the middle of the message.

   C. Listener modifying what he or she hears so that it conforms to the listener's expectations.

   D. Feeling uncomfortable hearing a patient talk about dying.

   E. Being concerned that the patient will not accept you as a "real" nurse."

   F. Being embarrassed when a client discusses his or her sexual problems.

      1. alienation from communication
      2. message anxiety
      3. human error in the communication process

7. Why is it important for nurses to be good listeners? Fill in the blanks with one of the choices given below:

   The nurse-client relationship is A. ________________, and meaningful

   B. ________________ requires C. ________________ listening.

   A. 1. intrapersonal
      2. interpersonal
      3. extrapersonal

   B. 1. reaction
      2. talking
      3. interaction

   C. 1. selective
      2. effective
      3. passive

8. Which of the following are *not* specific benefits of active listening?

   A. continuous observation of client

   B. "fuel" for effective interaction

   C. support of client

   D. listener can "round off" messages

   E. diagnostic tool for planning care

   F. message can be "filtered"

   G. therapeutic relationship

   H. learning by client *and* nurse

   I. agreement with listener's opinions

   J. listener can judge speaker

9. True (T) or False (F)?

   ______ A. Effective listening is simple to learn since poor listening habits are easily corrected.

   ______ B. It is sometimes helpful to preface your feedback with phrases such as "You feel . . ." or "I hear you say . . ."

_____ C. Almost everyone is able to be direct when speaking or discussing concerns.

_____ D. If your feedback is not accepted by the speaker, you should explain why you thought it was what he or she meant.

_____ E. It is important that your feedback minimally disrupts the flow of the person to whom you are listening.

10. Match the guideline for listening (number) with the appropriate collection of ideas (letter). One of the numbered words is not a true guideline, and will not be used.

    A. Listen for basic message, restate a summary, and obtain confirmation fo accuracy and helpfulness.

    B. Reword what you heard, ask for confirmation about accuracy, and allow speaker to correct your misunderstanding.

    C. Admit confusion, and try a restatement or ask for repetition or illustration.

    D. Look at speaker, maintain relaxed posture, use natural gestures, and relate statements without interrupting, or presenting new topics.

    1. attending
    2. responding
    3. paraphrasing
    4. clarifying
    5. perception checking

Posttest Answers

---

1. C 2. D 3. D 4. A. 2 B. c C. 1 D. 3 E. 2 F. 1
5. B 6. A. 1 B. 3 C. 3 D. 2 E. 1 F. 2 7. A. 2–interpersonal
B. 3–interaction C. 2–effective 8. D, F, I. J 9. A. False b. True
C. False D. False E. True 10. A. 3 B. 5 C. 4 D. 1

REFERENCES

1. Brammer, Lawrence M. *The Helping Relationship* Englewood Cliffs, New Jersey: Prentice-Hall, Inc., 1973), pp. 81-87.

2. Egan, Gerard, *Encounter: Group Processes for Interpersonal Growth* (Belmont, California: Brooks/Cole Publishing Co., 1970), pp. 248-260.

3. Lewis, Garland K. *Nurse-Patient Communication* (Dubuque, Iowa: Wm. C. Brown Co., 1973), pp. 35-44.

4. O'Brien, Maureen J. *Communications and Relationships in Nursing* (St. Louis: C.V. Mosby Co., 1974), pp. 33-39.

Feedback

DIRECTIONS

1. Complete the pretest. If you answer all the questions correctly, you may choose to complete the unit on feedback for added enrichment and knowledge.
2. After the pretest, complete the activities as directed. The activities and exercises should be completed in the order presented.
3. In order to complete the unit, you will need a pencil or pen. No other materials are needed.
4. A posttest will be given at the end of the unit. Successful completion of this test is necessary for you to have met the unit objectives.

OBJECTIVES

Upon completion of this unit on feedback, the learner will be able to:

1. Define feedback.
2. Describe the feedback process.
3. List and explain three sources of feedback.
4. Recognize three influences on giving and receiving feedback.
5. Identify five kinds of feedback.
6. Discuss the results of feedback.
7. Formulate a criteria for effective feedback.
8. Select ten examples of feedback and evaluate them as to appropriateness.

Pretest

Circle the correct answers.

1. All of the following phrases define feedback except:

   A. the return to you of behavior you have generated

   B. a regulatory (checks and balance) mechanism in communication

   C. the act of altering the sender's message until it meets the expectation of the receiver

   D. a process of checking out if message sent is message received and vice versa

2. Which of the following is not considered part of the feedback process?

   A. perceiving (receiving)

   B. assuming (internal validation)

   C. reacting (coding)

   D. responding (sending)

3. In communication, feedback is usually one way. T F

4. A person often gives feedback to himself. T F

5. Looking in the mirror provides an individual with a reflection, but this would not be considered feedback. T F

6. The "Looking Glass Self" concept refers to the image one sees when looking in the mirror. T F

7. Interpersonal interaction almost always includes feedback exchange.
   T F

8. Which of the following will most likely influence feedback exchange?

   A. relationship

   B. socioeconomic level

   C. expectations

   D. all of the above

   E. none of the above

9. All of the following are considered kinds of feedback except:

   A. acknowledging

   B. validating

   C. responding

   D. clarifying

   E. extending

   F. altering

10. Circle any of the following which are *desired* results of effective feedback?

    A. acceptance

    B. rejection

    C. rationalization

    D. displacement

    E. aborted interaction

    F. defensive reaction

11. Circle any of the following characteristics which make feedback *in-effective.*

    A. immediate
    B. negative
    C. destructive
    D. specific
    E. constructive
    F. positive
    G. delayed
    H. vague

12. Which of the following would be considered *appropriate* feedback?

    A. A *smile* in response to a friend saying, "You make me angry."

    B. *Congratulating* a friend who has just won a scholarship.

    C. *Critique* of fellow student who just practiced a speech for your reaction.

    D. *Shaming* a child you have discovered masturbating.

    E. *Reassuring* a friend that he or she will pass an exam when the friend tells you that he or she hasn't studied.

    F. *Staring* at a teacher who has said, "Watch me while I demonstrate."

    G. *Punishing* a friend with silence after he or she has hurt your feelings.

    H. *Empathisizing* with a friend who said, "I don't trust people who cheat on exams."

    I. *Frowning* when you have been censured for running a red light.

    J. *Complimenting* a friend on his ability to break the rules without getting caught.

Pretest Answers

1. C 2. B 3. F 4. T 5. F 6. F 7. T 8. D
9. C 10. A only 11. B, C, G, H 12. B, C, F, H, I

INTRODUCTION

For a definition of feedback, Luft states, "In its simplest sense, feedback refers to the return to you of behavior you have generated" (4:116). Another way of describing feedback is as a process of checking out if the message sent is the message received and vice versa. A simple model for communication illustrates that feedback serves as a regulatory (checks and balance) mechanism.

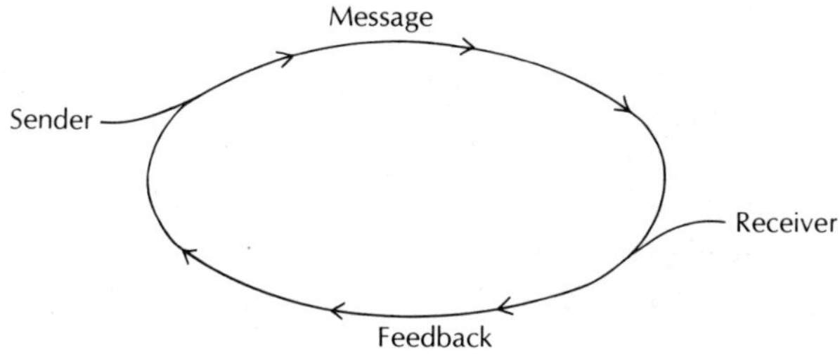

FEEDBACK: A DYNAMIC PROCESS

Feedback is a dynamic process and includes: (1) perceiving (receiving); (2) reacting (coding); and (3) responding (sending). The process is circular in that it almost always repeats itself in a cycle of giving-receiving-giving and so on. Trace the process in the following poem.

Cycles In My Life

I feel rejection
    which brings
Feelings of worthlessness
    which brings
Self-hate
    which makes me
Seek escape by
    hiding from others
    refusing to share
    becoming defensive

which causes
Others to react against my defenses
which brings on
Further feelings of
Rejection
which starts the cycle again.

I trust myself as
worthwhile
having something to offer
which causes me to
Affirm myself
which enables me to
Open myself and
share with others
who respond with
Love and acceptance
which verifies
My self-worth
which inspires me to
Trust myself
And the cycle starts all over again.

MAXIE DUNNAM
Dancing At My Funeral

Refer to the communication model and the feedback process, and answer the following questions about the poem:

1. What message is being sent in each cycle?
2. What is the receiver likely perceiving in each cycle?
3. What reacting by the receiver is probable in each cycle?
4. What feedback message might the receiver send back to the sender in each cycle?

Response:

Cycle I

1. I don't like you. I am angry, and so on.

2. He or she doesn't like me. He or she is angry, and so on.
3. I don't like people who don't like me. I don't like people who are angry.
4. Go away, I don't like you. Go away, I'm angry with you.

Cycle II

1. I want to share with you because I like you.
2. He or she is friendly and likes me.
3. I will be friendly with that person. I like him or her.
4. I like you. You are a nice person.

Feedback often is intrapsychic and intrapersonal. Answer for yourself the question, "How do I feel?"

I feel

This is an example of internal feedback. A mirror represents an external source of feedback, but it is also intrapersonal. What feedback might you give yourself if you saw your reflection and wanted to check out your hair?

My hair is

External feedback is that which one gets from outside sources—people (interpersonal), animals, even inanimate objects. Examples of this might be:

1. A friend telling you, "Hey, you look great today!"
2. A kitten purring in response to your scratching its head, which says, "I like what you're doing."
3. A warm, soft bed feeling very comfortable, which says, "You are tired. You need rest."
4. An oral thermometer registering 98.6°, which says, "Your body temperature is normal."

Interpersonal feedback (from other people) contributes to the development of the "Looking Glass Self," the concept of self presented to the world that is based on how others react to, and evaluate, one's behavior. Respond to the following:

1. If several friends told me they did not like my talking so much I would see myself as
2. If people told me they liked my friendly attitude, I would see myself as

In her book, Lewis states that the giving and/or receiving of feedback may be influenced by several factors (Lewis, 1973, p. 79). Specifically she describes:

1. relationship
2. self-concept
3. socioeconomic level
4. education level
5. expectation

List four other common identifying features of an individual that might influence his or her giving/receiving feedback.

1.
2.
3.
4.

Possible responses are:

1. age
2. sex
3. race/ethnic group
4. health status

What five characteristics of yourself most influence your receiving and giving feedback?

1.
2.
3.
4.
5.

When (in what situations, with whom) do you find yourself comfortable in the feedback process? I feel comfortable in giving/receiving feedback when

Uncomfortable? I feel uncomfortable giving/receiving feedback when

Feedback can enhance your control of communication and interper--sonal relationships through your incorporating information about effects of your behavior, and it also is part of a steering device by which you can guage your reactions. "Acceptable" social communication often makes giving and receiving feedback difficult; therefore, many people get little idea of how they are coming across to others. Feedback then is a vital component of "professional" communication, and you can use it to help your clients and others improve their self-concept and to grow. Carter (1970) describes five types of feedback: (1) acknowledging; (2) validating; (3) clarifying; (4) extending; and (5) altering. The following are descriptions and examples of each type. The sender's message is, "My, it's hot in this room."

1. *Acknowledging.* This type of feedback simply acknowledges reception of the sender's message, for example, "I heard you say it's hot in here."
2. *Validating.* This type verifies the *accuracy* of the sender's message, for example, "Yes, you're right. It is hot in here." When perceptions are agreed with, the process is referred to as *consensual validation.*

3. *Clarifying.* This feedback verifies the *meaning* of the sender's message by checking out the receiver's comprehension of the sender's intent, for example, "Do you mean that you would like for me to open the window?"

4. *Extending.* This type of feedback adds to the sender's original message and enlarges its meaning, for example, "You feel hot because you're running a fever."

5. *Altering.* This type corrects or changes the sender's message, for example, "Actually it's only 62 degrees, so it's not hot at all. It must be that you are feeling hot."

Each of these five types sends a response that helps the sender to "keep on course" or else helps him or her to alter (correct) a course, which demonstrates that feedback is an essential part of nursing. Practice using each kind of feedback to respond to others. You will be successful when you can easily respond to any message with one of the five types of feedback.

Utilizing each kind of feedback, write a response to the statement made by a friend, "That exam was really hard!"

1. Acknowledging:

2. Validating:

3. Clarifying:

4. Extending:

5. Altering:

Possible answers are:

1. You found the test difficult.
2. You're right. It was a lulu!

3. Are you concerned whether you passed it?
4. Do you think your grade for the course is in jeopardy?
5. I found the test easy. Did you study for it?

How might you, as a nurse, respond to a patient who stated, "That pill made me sick to my stomach."

1. Acknowledging:

2. Validating:

3. Clarifying:

4. Extending:

5. Altering:

Possible responses are:

1. The medication made you nauseated.
2. That medication has that side affect.
3. Are you saying you don't want to take the medication?
4. Is this the first time the medication has affected you this way?
5. I'm fairly certain your nausea is due to the lab procedure, not the medication.

As a review activity, complete the following puzzle. Fill in the blanks, using the statements numbered 1 through 8 following the puzzle. The solution appears at the end of the presentation.

1. _ _ _ _ _ _ f _ _ _ _

2. _ e _ _ _ _ _ _ _

3. e _ _ _ _ _ _ _ _

4. _ _ _ _ d _ _ _ _ _ _

5. b _ _ _ _ _ _ _

6. a _ _ _ _ _ _ _

7. _ _ _ c _ _ _ _ _ _

8. _ _ k _ _ _ _ _ _ _ _ _ _

1. This type of feedback verifies the *meaning* of the sender's message.
2. This step in the feedback process is also known as coding.
3. This type of feedback adds to the sender's original message and enlarges its meaning.
4. This type of feedback verifies the *accuracy* of the sender's message.
5. Feedback is the return to you of ____________ you have generated.
6. This type of feedback corrects or changes the sender's message.
7. This step in the feedback process is also known as receiving.
8. This type of feedback indicates reception of the sender's message.
9. The step in the feedback process that was left out was ____________.

Depending on a variety of factors, feedback may be accepted or rejected. It may also be rationalized, or a defensive reaction may occur. Other possible results include displacement of elicited feelings, or more obvious, an aborted interaction. Factors that might affect the result of feedback are: (1) need; (2) energy level; (3) emotional state; (4) timing; and (5) situation. For optimal effectiveness, feedback should be:

1. immediate
2. specific
3. constructive
4. positive

as opposed to:

1. delayed
2. vague
3. destructive
4. negative

In utilizing this criteria, it is important to differentiate between the *social* definition of positive/negative and that of systems theory. In systems theory, positive feedback is that which enhances growth or development. Negative feedback, on the other hand, inhibits or blocks movement of the system. Thus, it is not always effective to give *socially* positive feedback. What might result if a friend told you, "You look really nice," if you knew your appearance was unkempt or sloppy? What would happen to your intrapersonal and interpersonal systems? Would it be effective for a nurse to tell a client, "No one will even notice that you have no legs."? Give a *more positive* response to a client's statement, "I feel self-conscious about having no legs."

1. Acknowledging:

2. Validating:

3. Clarifying:

4. Extending:

5. Altering:

Possible answers:

1. You feel self-conscious about your legs.
2. You see yourself as being different from others.
3. Do you think people will tend to pity you?
4. Are you concerned about how you will be able to get around?
5. From our conversation earlier, my hunch is that you're more concerned about what your wife will think of you.

As a Big Finish to this module, complete the following crossword puzzle. All of the words are examples of verbal and nonverbal feedback from common, day-to-day interactions. As you fill in the words, consider when each would be appropriate and when inappropriate.

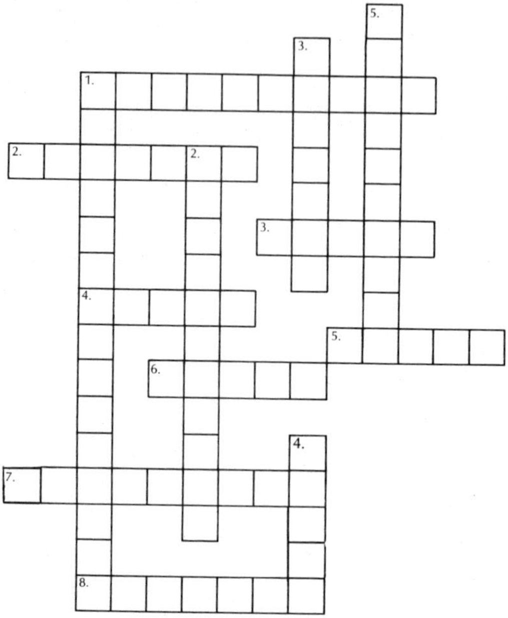

Across

1. A formal act of courtesy; something said in praise.
2. A blaming; condemnation.
3. To cause to feel dishonor or disgrace.
4. Firm belief in the honesty, reliability, and so on of another; faith.
5. To gaze steadily and intently.
6. To contract the brows, as in displeasure or concentration.
7. The act of making judgments; a finding fault.
8. A keeping still; absence of sound or noise.

Down

1. Expressions of pleasure over another's good fortune or accomplishment.
2. Assuring again; restoring to confidence.
3. Intellectual or emotional identification with another.
4. To show pleasure, amusement, affection, etc. by an upward curving of the mouth.
5. A penalty imposed to cause pain, loss, etc, as for a crime.

The solution is at the end of the presentation.

Now that you have finished the module, let me leave you with this classic illustration of feedback. Read it carefully—it really does make sense.

> I know you believe you understand what you think I said, but I am not sure you realize that what you heard is not what I meant.

Now do the posttest and check your answers. Thank you for your attention and participation. I wish you success in giving and receiving much positive feedback.

Puzzle Answers

Page 116 1. clarifying 2. reacting 3. extending 4. validating 5. behavior 6. altering 7. perceiving 8. acknowledging 9. responding (sending).

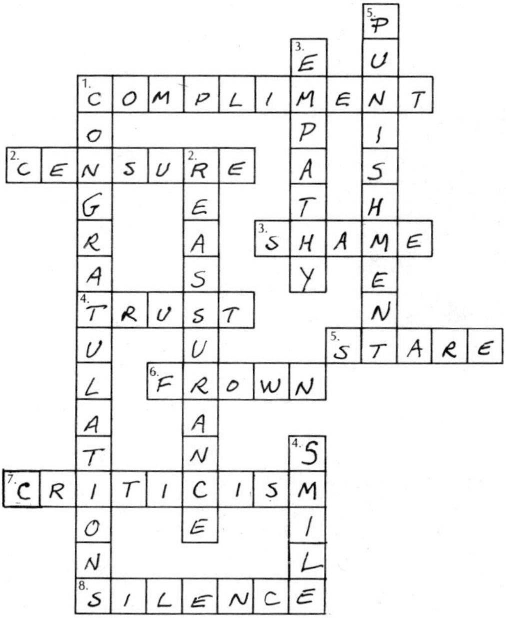

Posttest

1. Write a definition of feedback. Feedback is:

2. List the three components of the feedback process.

   A.

   B.

   C.

3. List three sources of feedback.

   A.

   B.

   C.

4. Which of the following will likely influence feedback exchange?

   A. self-concept

   B. socioeconomic level

   C. educational level

   D. all of the above

   E. none of the above

5. List the five types of feedback.

   A.

   B.

   C.

   D.

   E.

6. Which of the following would *not* affect the result of feedback?

   A. need and energy

   B. emotional state

   C. timing and situation

   D. all of the above

   E. none of the above

7. For optimal effectiveness, feedback should be:

   A.

   B.

   C.

   D.

8. Which of the following would be considered *appropriate* feedback?

   A. A smile in response to a friend saying, "You make me angry."

   B. Congratulating a friend who has just won a scholarship.

   C. Criticism of a fellow student who just practiced a speech for your reaction.

   D. Shaming a child you have discovered masturbating.

   E. Reassuring a friend that he or she will pass an exam when the friend tells you that he or she has not studied.

   F. Staring at a teacher who has said, "Watch me while I demonstrate."

G. Punishing a friend with silence after he or she has hurt your feelings.

H. Empathizing with a friend who said, "I don't trust people who cheat."

I. Frowning when you have been censured for running a red light.

J. Complimenting a friend on his or her ability to break the rules without getting caught.

Posttest Answers

1. The return to you of behavior you have generated, or, A process of checking out if the message sent is the message received, or, A regulatory (checks and balances) mechanism in communication that is cyclical.
2. A. perceiving (receiving) B. reacting (coding) C. responding (sending)
3. A. self B. a mirror C. other people D. animals E. objects
4. D
5. A. acknowledging B. validating C. clarifying D. extending E. altering
6. E
7. A. immediate B. specific C. constructive D. positive
8. B C F H I

REFERENCES

1. Carter, Ruth. *Communication Exercises* (San Jose State University, Department of Nursing, San Jose, California, 1970).

2. Egan, Gerard, *Encounter: Group Processes for Interpersonal Growth* (Belmont, California: Brooks/Cole Publishing Co., 1970).

3. Lewis, Garland. *Nurse-Patient Communication* (Dubuque, Iowa: Wm. C. Brown Co., 1973), pp. 78–81.

4. Luft, Joseph. *Of Human Interaction* (Palo Alto, California: National Press Books, 1969).

Body Language

DIRECTIONS

1. Complete the pretest. If you answer all the questions correctly, you may choose to complete the unit on body language for added enrichment and knowledge.
2. After the pretest, complete the activities as directed. The activities and exercises should be completed in the order presented.
3. In order to complete the unit, you will need a pencil or pen. No other materials are needed.
4. A posttest will be given at the end of the unit. Successful completion of this test is necessary for you to have met the unit objectives.

OBJECTIVES

Upon completion of this unit on body language, the learner will be able to:

1. List three variables that influence body language.
2. Select four variables that qualify messages.
3. Define "points" in body language.
4. Describe at least three different points and their common meanings.
5. Describe what a change in position may mean during a conversation.
6. Define "presentation" in body language.
7. List at least three variables that determine social distance during a conversation.
8. Describe how status affects the way in which one approaches someone sitting at a desk.
9. List two grooming mannerisms for men and two for women.
10. Describe at least four common body language messages sent by clients to nurses.

Pretest

1. Body language is influenced by all of the following *except:*

    A. social class

    B. personal style

    C. genetic characteristics

    D. ethnic background

2. The messages from one person to another are qualified by all of the following *except:*

    A. educational background

    B. verbal content

    C. vocal and linguistic patterns

    D. body movement

3. Movements of the head, face and hands are referred to as in body language.

    A. mannerisms

    B. styles

    C. kinesics

    D. points

4. In most conversations, eye contact lasts about ________ seconds before one or both persons look away.

   A. 1

   B. 5

   C. 10

   D. 15

5. The pupils of the eye are most likely to dilate when the person views a situation that is:

   A. pleasant

   B. stressful

   C. anxious

   D. intense

6. Rubbing the eye is generally considered a way of expressing:

   A. seriousness

   B. lack of acceptance

   C. indifference

   D. lack of understanding

7. The part of our body that we frequently conceal is/are:

   A. face

   B. hands

   C. torso

   D. legs

8. A sequence of several points is called a ________________ in body language.

   A. posture

   B. position

   C. presentation

   D. penetration

9. A shift in position tells us all of the following *except:*

   A. what is happening

   B. that something is happening

   C. an emotional state is involved

   D. something about attitude

10. Relaxation is a good indicator of:

    A. comfort

    B. alertness

    C. status

    D. performance

11. The territory two people establish between themselves in a conversation is affected by:

    A. level of intimacy

    B. ethnicity

    C. the business they have together

    D. all of these

    E. none of these

12. Incongruent posture in a conversation usually indicates:

    A. confusion

    B. boredom

    C. disagreement

    D. relaxation

13. Grooming mannerisms that relate to sexuality are all of the following *except:*

    A. influenced by the culture

    B. made with risk of rejection

    C. usually made by women

    D. affected by the timing

14. When a client turns away from the nurse, the person is most likely to be expressing any of the following *except:*

    A. boredom

    B. isolation

    C. anger

    D. sadness

Pretest Answers

1. C 2. A 3. D 4. A 5. A 6. B 7. D 8. B 9. A 10. C
11. D 12. C 13. C 14. A

INTRODUCTION

When we are conversing with someone, and they look at us attentively, seem relaxed, and maintain a close but comfortable distance, we feel at ease and understood. Conversely, when our conversational partner does not maintain eye contact, has a rigid posture, and sits far away, we feel uncomfortable. It is very important for us to use and understand body language so that we will become more effective communicators, personally and professionally.

This module consists of slides and/or photographs, and a printed script that discusses the major components of body language. The photographs are mostly of persons in everyday activities but the principles apply equally to clients, colleagues, and family members.

It is important to know at the beginning that this module refers to common meanings of body language. Since many variables are involved in all the conversations we participate in, be certain to validate your meanings with the persons concerned. If it is not appropriate or convenient to validate your inferences about body language, at least remember that you *are* making an inference.

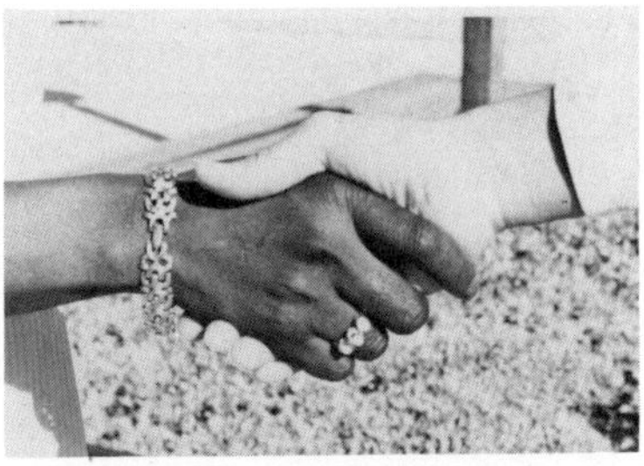

Hi, welcome to body language module.

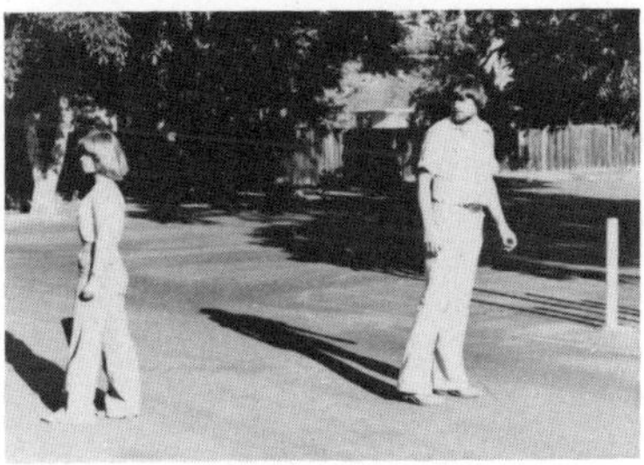

Every culture has a particular body language. It is influenced by ethnic background, social class, and personal style. Once you learn how to read it, and you often do so unconsciously, the messages are quite clear.

All movements of the body have meaning, whether the setting is in a hospital or in the home. In addition, body language may be significant in one context and not in another.

The messages from one person to another are qualified by:

1. *the context in which they take place*
2. *verbal context*
3. *vocal and linguistic patterns*
4. *body movements.*

Many times what we think is intuition is a careful reading of these variables, particularly body movements.

The technical term for body language is kinesics, *the study of communication through body movements.*

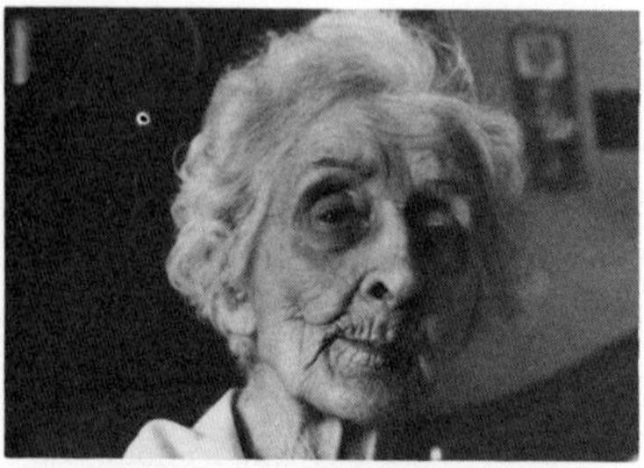

Movements of the head, face, and hands are referred to as points *in body language. There are as many as 135 points of the head, face, and hands. When you consider the endless combinations that are possible, it is easy to understand the complexity of body language. Even increasing our perception of a few points will lead to better observation skills.*

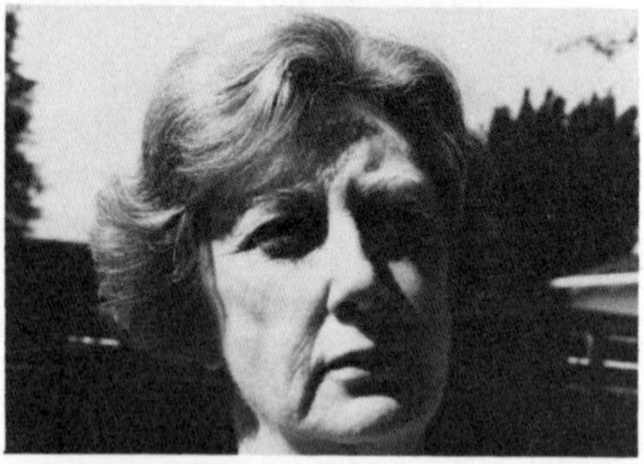

Points related to the eyes are of great interest to most of us. Eyes are frequently described as steely-knowing-mocking-piercing-glowing, when in fact, the eyes reveal very little without the face around them. In this picture the eye points cannot be separated from the forehead, eyebrow, and mouth points.

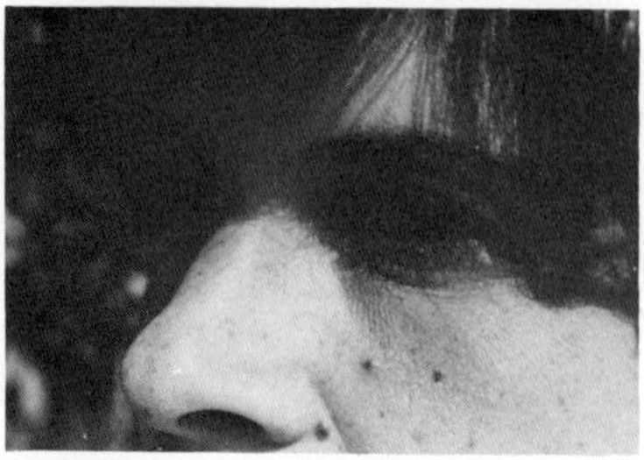

In most circumstances eye contact lasts about a second before one or both persons look away. If we like someone we tend to look a little longer than usual. People who maintain eye contact are usually considered to be sending messages of interest, sincerity, and self-confidence. Ask a colleague to time your eye contact with three different clients. A second can be timed by counting, "one thousand one, one thousand two," and so on.

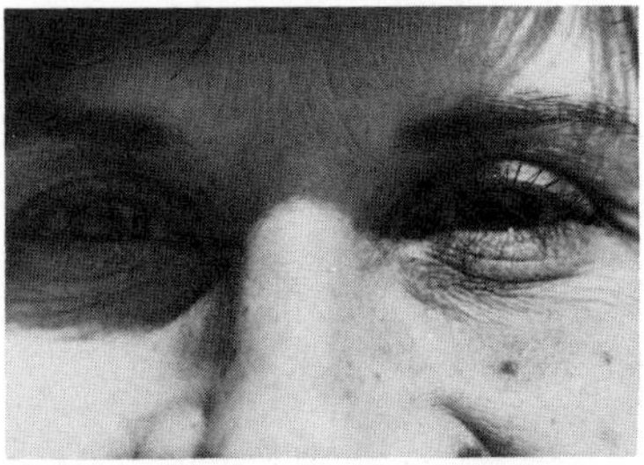

Longer looks or stares are considered an invasion of privacy. Even when the stare is accompanied by other pleasant points, most people become quite anxious when they are watched intently. When we are caught sneaking a glance at someone we tend to send other body messages that say, "Oops, it was an accident."

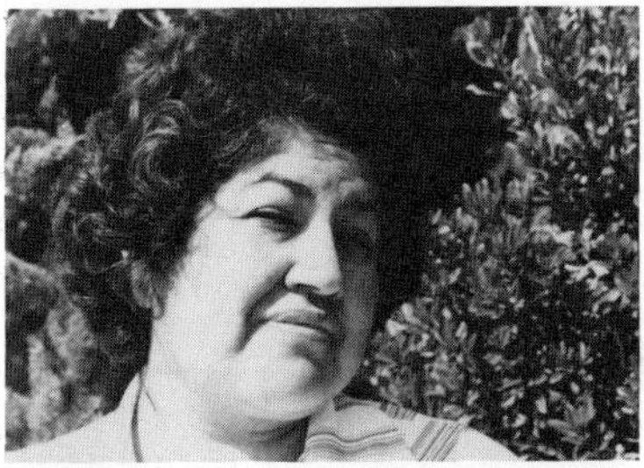

Stares may be used to convey a put down message, they are also used to send sexual messages. Because of the accompanying body language we usually read the stare correctly.

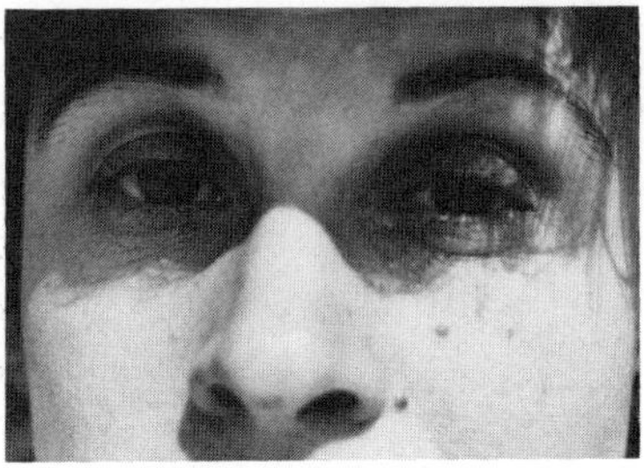

Most of our expressions last one half second to a second but they can also be as rapid as 1/150 of a second. This indicates the importance of maintaining eye contact with a person you are interviewing or assessing.

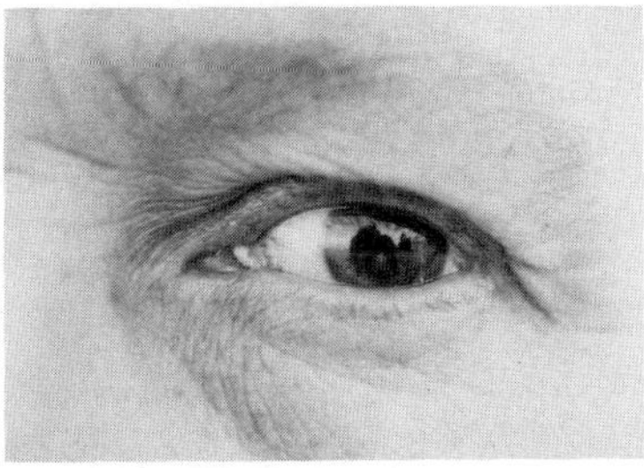

Experiments have demonstrated a relationship between the size of a person's pupils and emotions. The pupils dilate when they see something pleasant. However, anxiety and intense interest can also cause enlargement of the pupils. The important thing to remember is that pupil dilation is a clue to internal responses. Consider for a moment how you could use this clue when talking to a client.

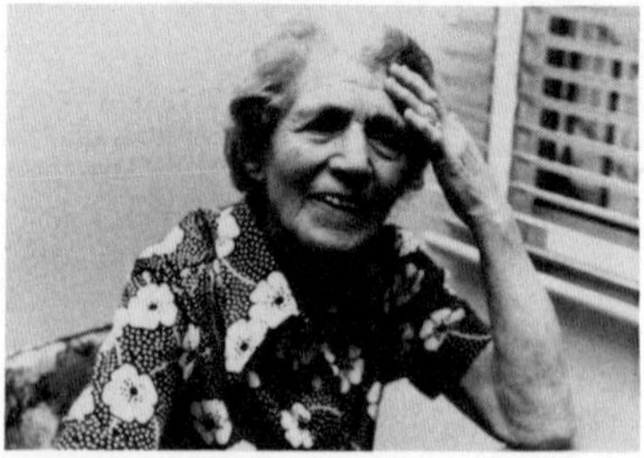

The eyebrows have over 23 possible positions. We ask a question with them, or express disbelief as demonstrated here. We flash them to express a greeting, show a joke, or suggest a sense of showing a common reaction to a situation.

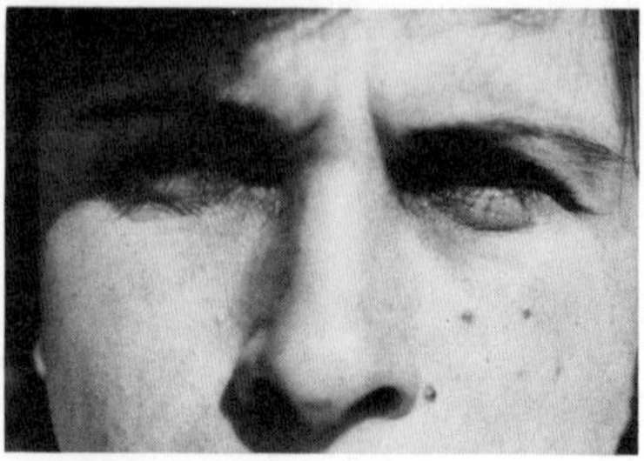

In an angry frown the eyebrows will be depressed on the inside as demonstrated here. In a sad frown the eyebrows will ordinarily be drawn at the outer ends.

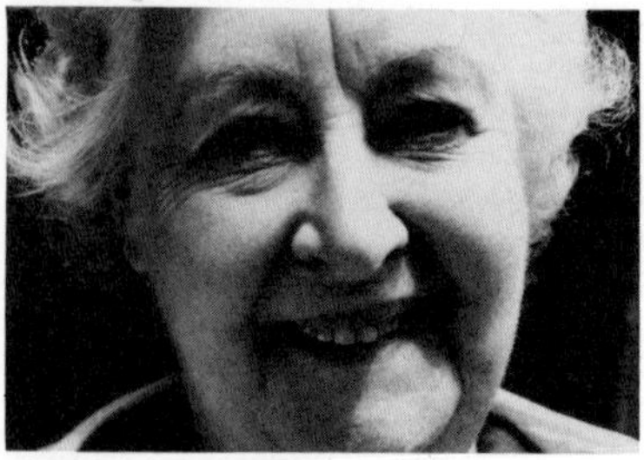

The smile is an upward and outward movement at the corners of the mouth. Although we generally want to see the expression of the eyes, eyebrows and forehead to interpret the smile message, as you can see the mouth alone is quite expressive.

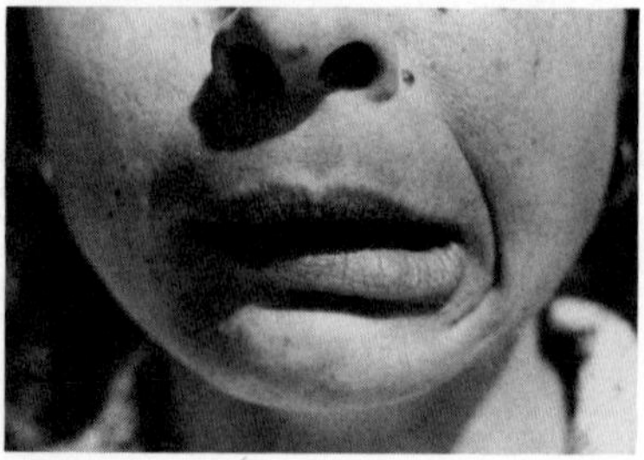

When the corners of the mouth are turned downward we usually read a message of sadness, anger or concern. Study the mouths of persons you know and consider if the typical expression of their mouth is consistent with their optimistic or pessimistic approach to life. Can you infer anything about a client's health by the position of the mouth? Keep your own record of the client's mouth points at the beginning of every day and then compare your findings with other data.

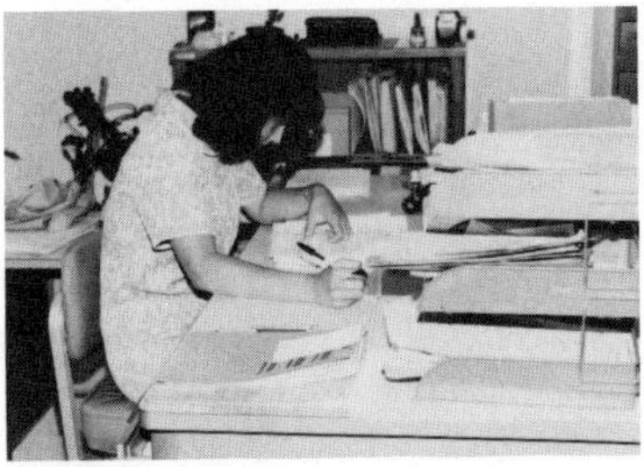

We depend on facial points to indicate our approach to others. Seriousness, for example, is indicated by holding very still, cocking the head slightly and looking intently at the speaker.

In addition, you may express seriousness by stroking your chin or carefully scratching your head.

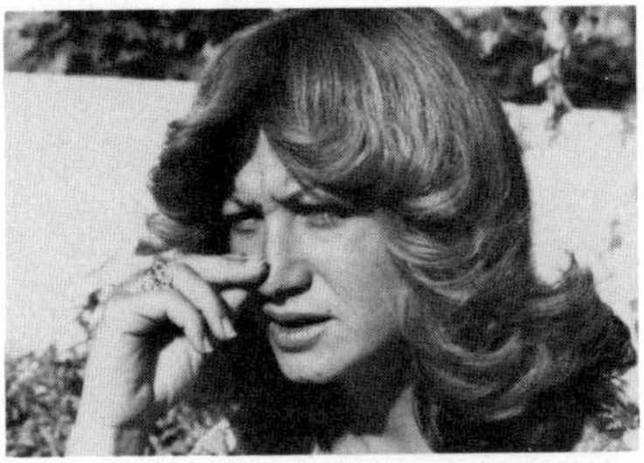

Rubbing the nose is done to indicate a negative evaluation or express puzzlement, or indicate a rule has been broken.

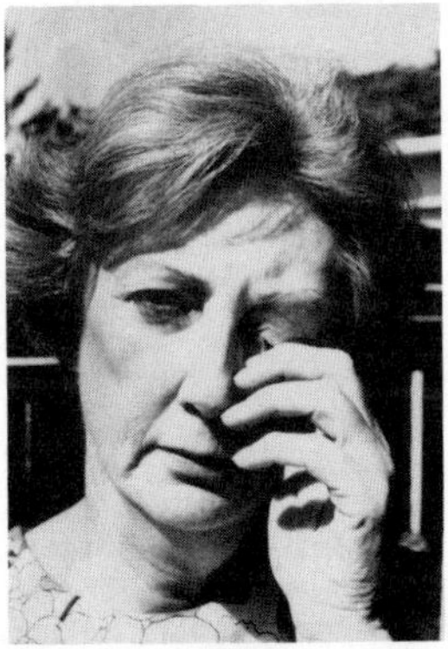

Rubbing the eye is often indicative of a refusal to accept something that is being pointed out by the speaker.

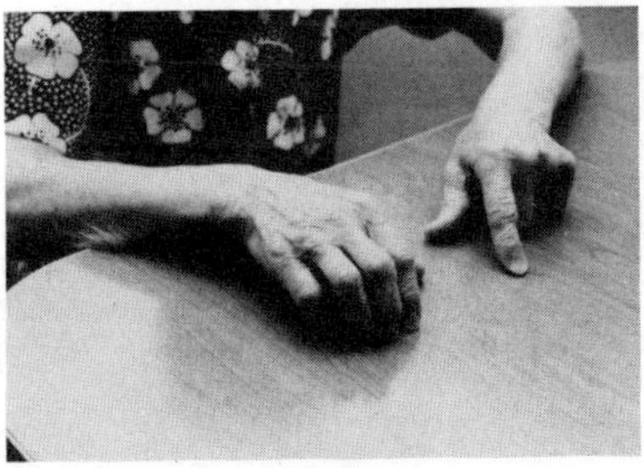

We tap our fingers to relate impatience. In a similar manner, we slap our forehead to indicate forgetfulness and shrug our shoulders to show indifference.

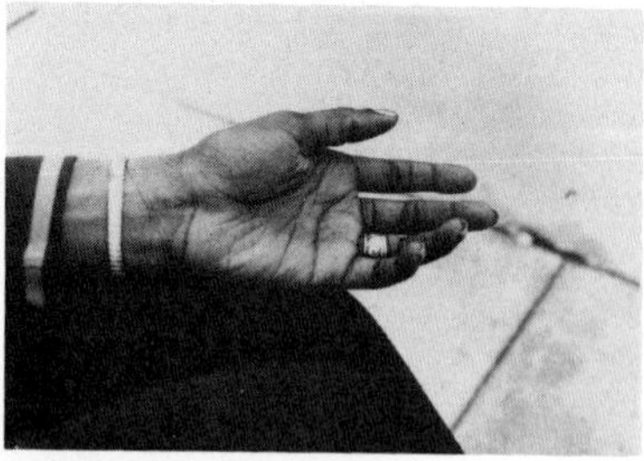

Hand points have many meanings. The open palm is a way of saying, "I'm being open with you." Research shows that we often unconsciously open our palm toward those who are threatening us verbally. When the hand is flat it can also send a message of, "I'm leveling with you."

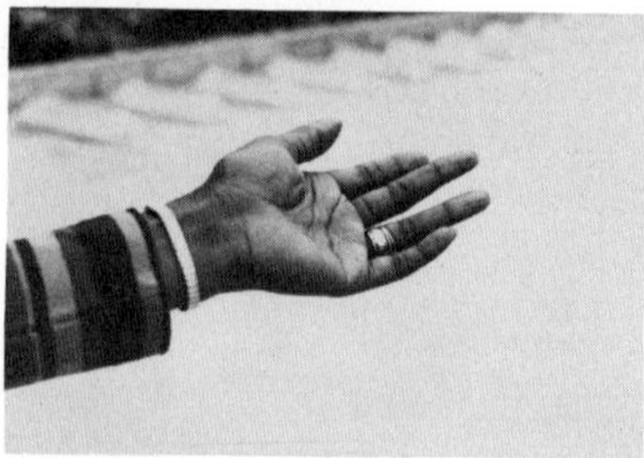

The outstretched hand is usually symbolically giving or taking. In this case it appears to be giving.

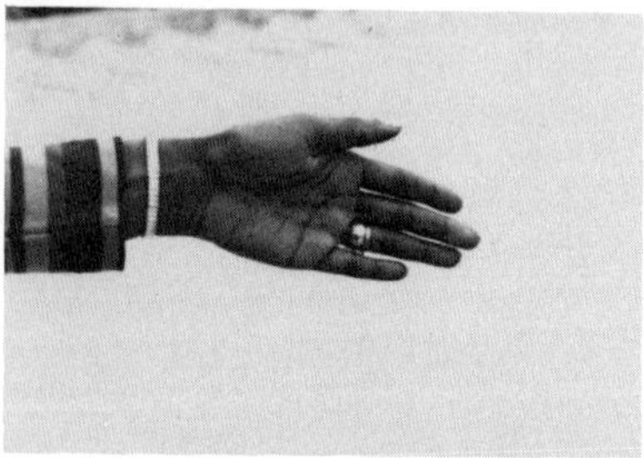

A cutting motion is used to express a desire to "chop off."

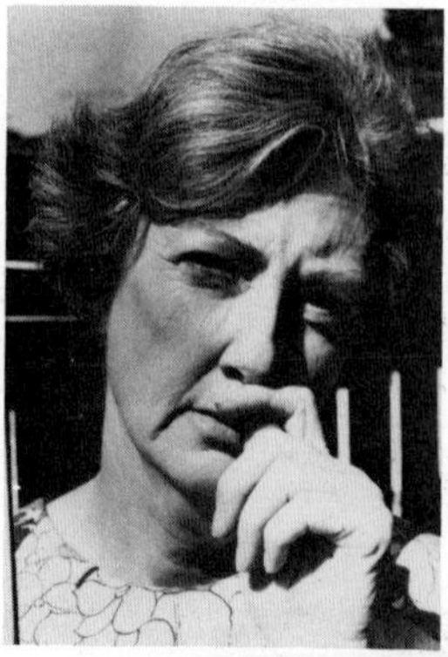

When we cover the mouth with our fingers or hand we are unconsciously telling ourself, "Keep the mouth shut." We could, of course, also be suggesting that the speaker quit talking or at least change the topic.

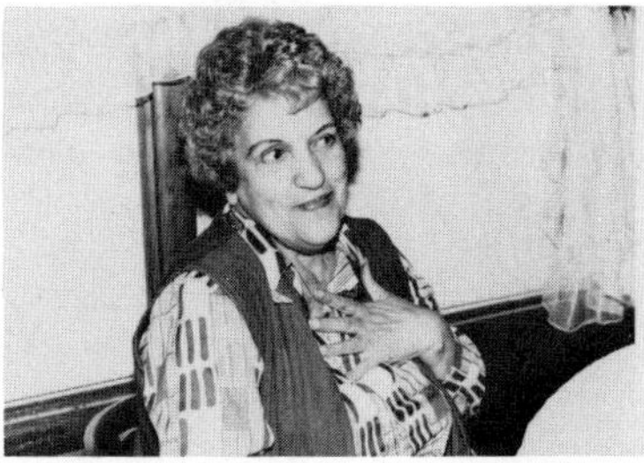

Placing the hand over the heart symbolizes loyalty and trustworthiness.

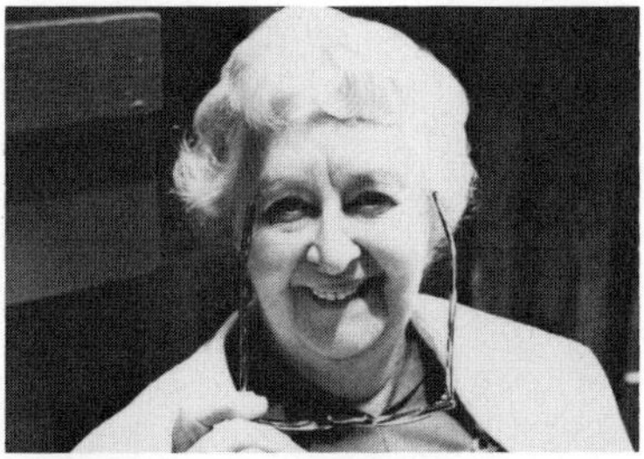

People who wear glasses often remove them to accentuate a point they are making.

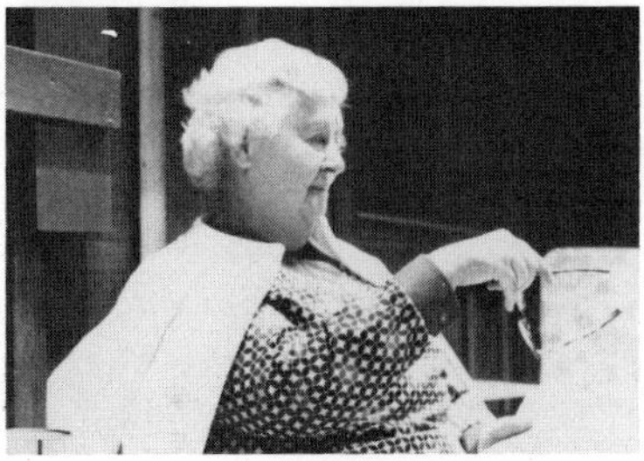

They also may remove their glasses to convey a message of disapproval or to question the status of another person.

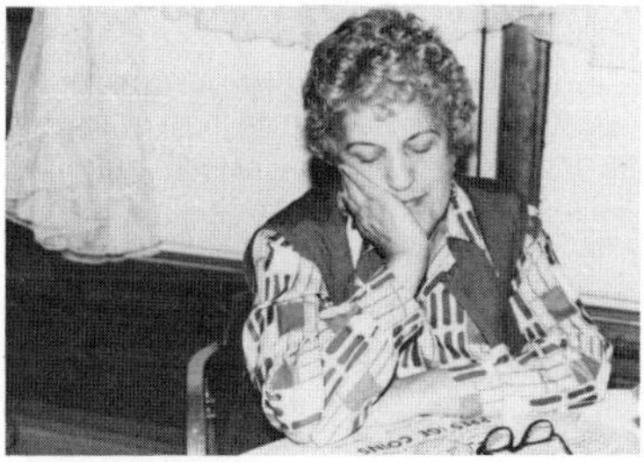

Resting the head upon the hand is an example of giving self-support. The support may be in response to a verbal threat or it may be support against boredom. It may also, of course, be just for comfort.

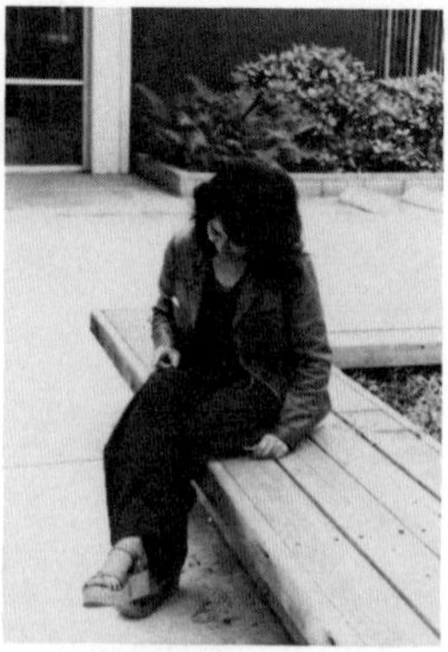

Flicking lint from clothes is frequently a response to a remark considered to be outrageous. It is also a response to suspicion. It can also just be a way to pass time.

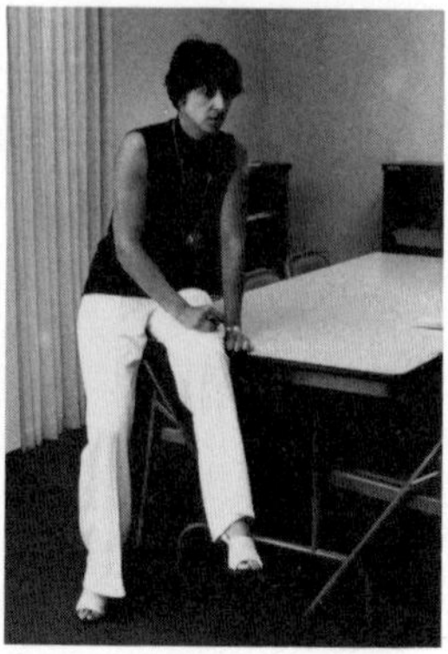

The legs and feet reveal anxiety and rage. Subtle leg movements are often made unconsciously. For example, many appear surprised when it is called to their attention that they have been swinging their leg during a period of anxiety. It has been noted that when people are being deceitful, they have fewer leg and foot movements than at other times. We often sit too closely to observe leg movements. We feel vulnerable when our legs are exposed and tend to protect them by sitting behind tables and desks.

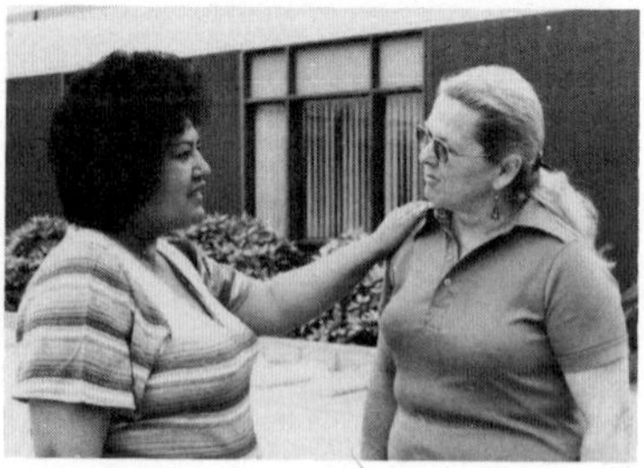

When there is a sequence of several points it is called a position. *A position is a postural shift involving at least half of the body. It can last for about five minutes on an average.*

We assume various positions for comfort and by habit. We also assume positions for particular purposes, such as we shift our position when we disagree with a speaker in preparation for delivering our protest, or to assume a new approach, or to indicate a desire to remove oneself from the communication.

A shift in position means that something is happening. It does not always tell us what is happening.

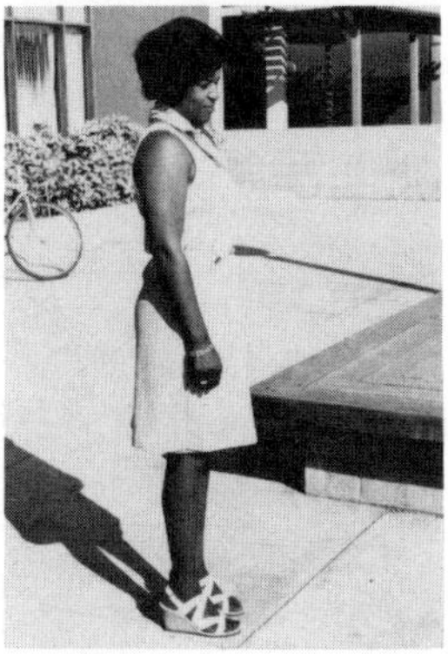

Different postures are related to different emotional states. We also use posture to indicate how we feel about ourselves and what our status is in the situation. Compare the postures of your three most recent clients and evaluate how their posture compared with the verbal messages they gave you.

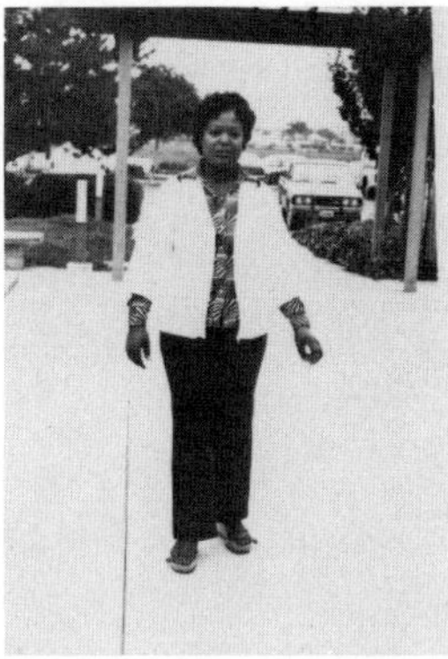

We generally think that the person with erect posture and squared shoulders is self-confident and responsible.

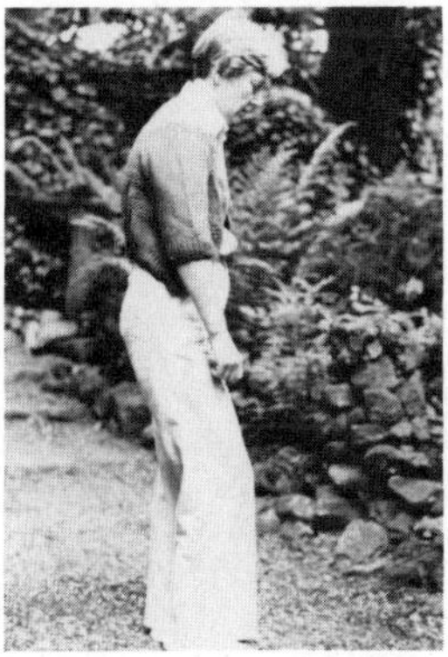

Walking in a slouch, however, with bowed shoulders indicates decreased self-confidence and indicates that the person is carrying a symbolic burden.

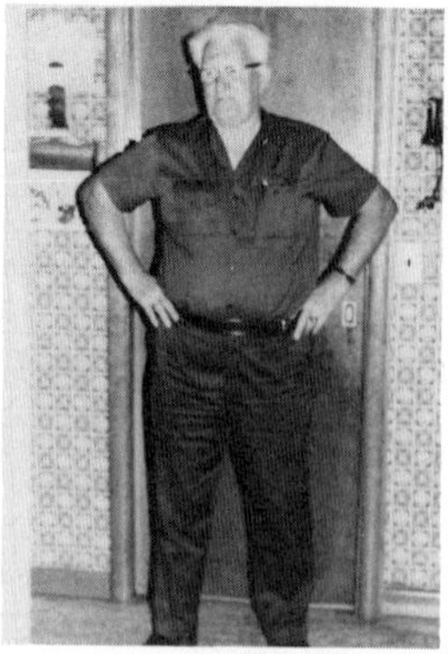

Standing erectly with hands on hips indicates authority and dominance, doesn't it?

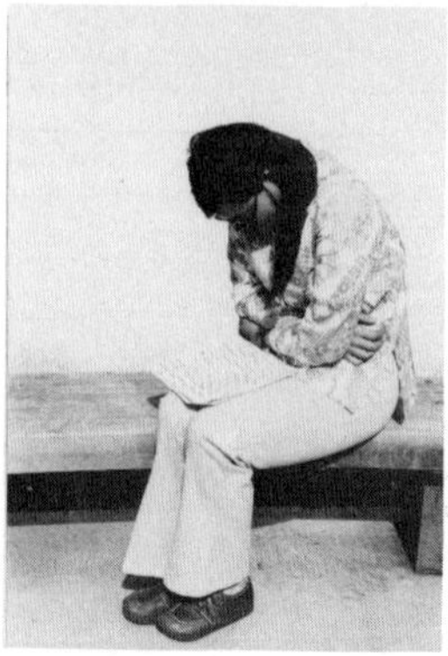

Sitting with shoulders curled inward portrays submissiveness and withdrawal.

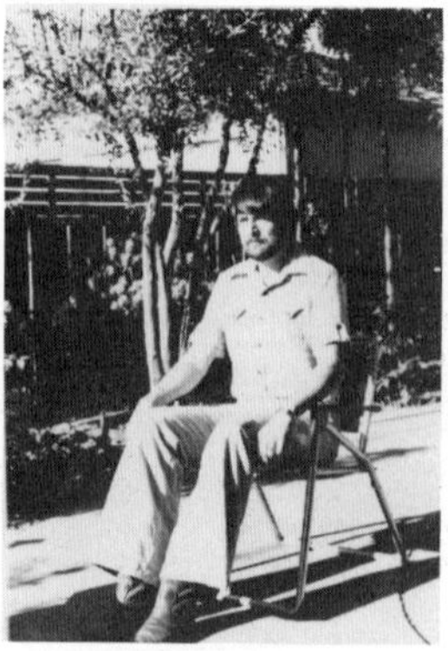

Relaxation of posture is a good indicator of both attitude and status. This man's erect posture indicates self-confidence and yet the rigidity of his position signifies he is not relaxed in this situation. Our posture is affected by whether we regard the other person as threatening.

When you can, assume the posture of your client and see if it gives you an idea of how that person may be feeling.

Observe the posture of others and determine if it is congruent with the conversation. Your posture often reflects your attitude toward the person you are with.

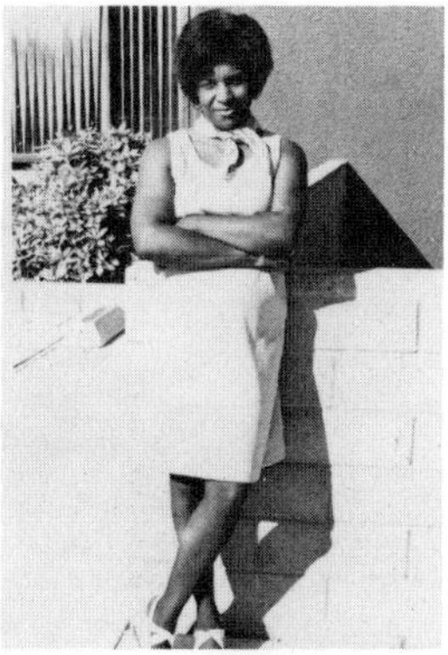

If you group together all the positions a person goes through in the course of a conversation you have a presentation. *A presentation can last up to several hours. It is terminated by a change in location.*

We also go through a presentation when we are done. For example, this woman presents herself as alone in a rather aggressive manner, indicated by her points and posture.

Clasping the arms and legs together may be done to protest or isolate the self.

We do assume presentation of isolation by leaning away from others and by turning away and placing a hand against our face as a shield.

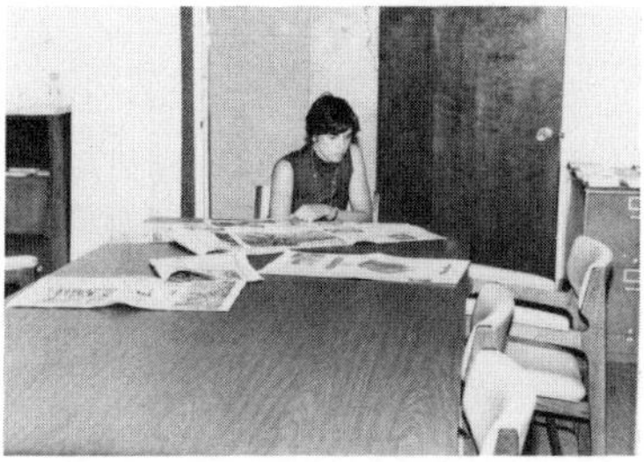

The person who wishes to sit alone will usually take a retreat position. She will usually take a table at the back of the room and face away from the door. She will sit at the corner of the table and indicate by her posture, "If you must sit here, leave me as much space as possible."

She may, however, as this woman does, sit aggressively at the center of the table and indicate by her body language, "This is my table, leave me alone."

Studies indicate that if body signals to be left alone are ignored, the person being invaded will move away.

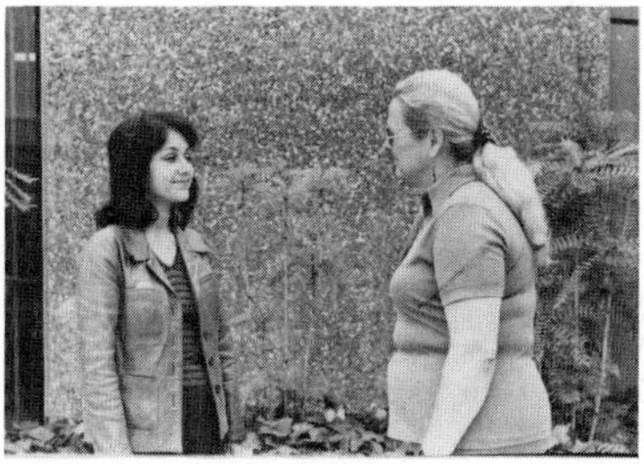

When two persons meet to converse they quickly establish a small territory of their own. They orient their bodies to each other, look at each other and establish a particular distance. Two people standing usually assume a distance of 24 inches. We usually stand just out of touch range and do not use much touch in a conversation. Are you comfortable with the distance you keep between you and your clients? Do you ever receive any body language that indicates you are too close or too far away?

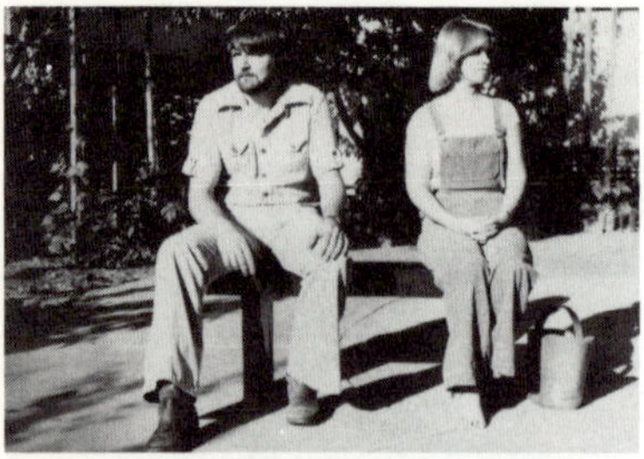

Two people sitting generally sit about 18 inches apart. The distance is determined by: (1) ethnicity; (2) level of intimacy; (3) prior relationship; (4) the business they have together; (5) available space; and (6) circumstances.

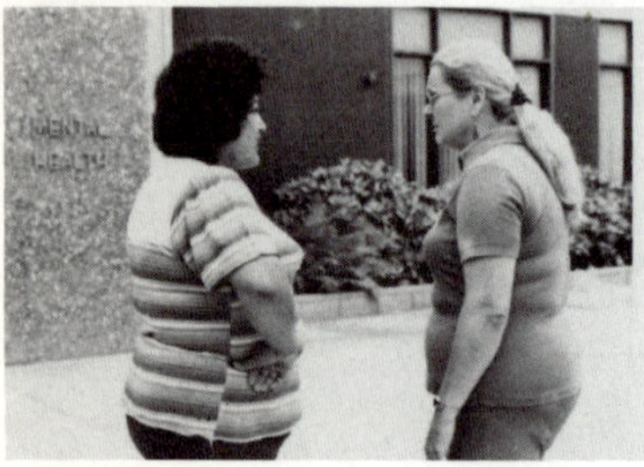

If the persons talking do not wish to be interrupted they will block others off by their positions. For example, they will turn face to face, stand closer together and turn an elbow out as a barrier. The legs may create barriers as well.

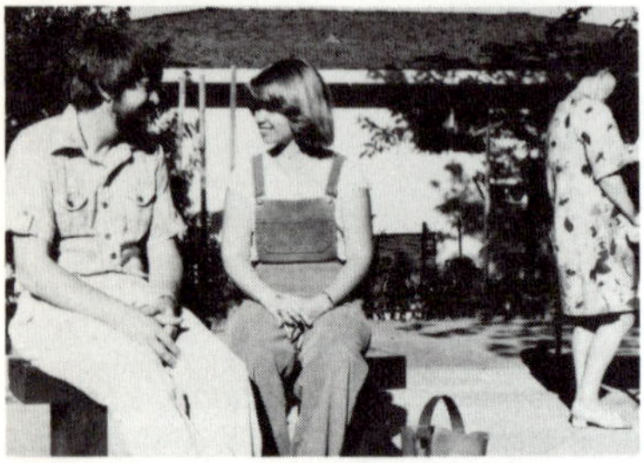

Generally we face each other to share feelings and thoughts or information. Sitting side by side is a more neutral position and prevents eye contact and observation of body language. How does communicating with a person in bed affect your communication?

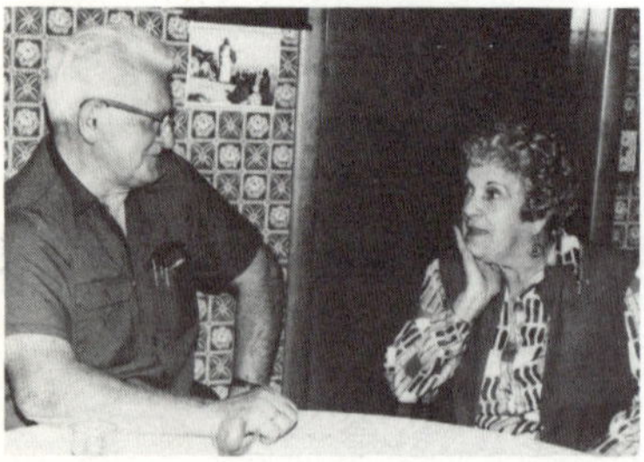

In this situation the participants are sitting face to face and in relaxed postures, however, the distance between them prevents an intimate conversation.

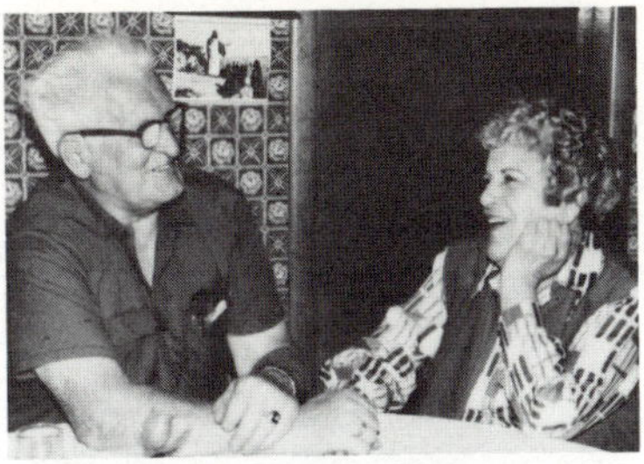

When we are involved in a conversation in which we share similar views, our postures are usually congruent.

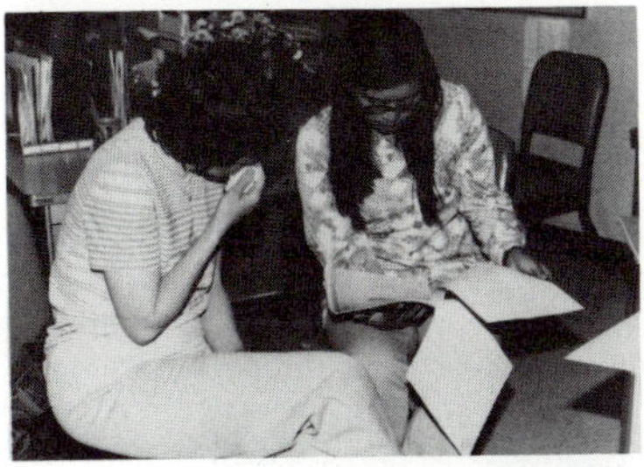

When a person wants to take a different position she often assumes a slightly incongruent position.

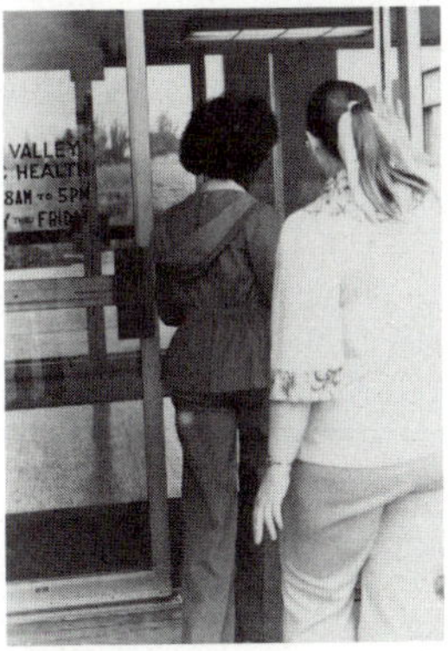

When people terminate a presentation, they discontinue their position. They step back, look down and away, turn out from each other and then leave.

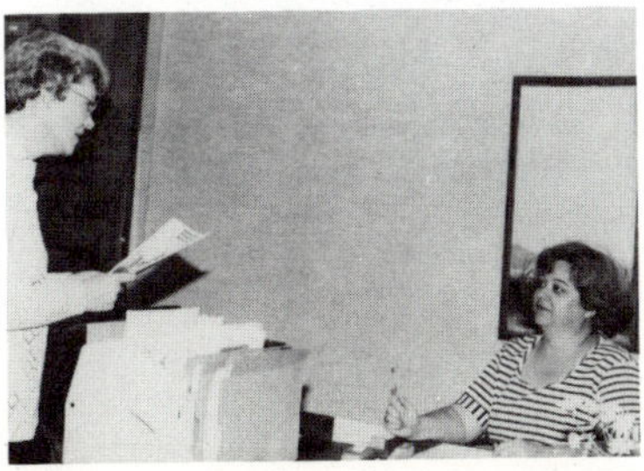

Our presentations are affected greatly by status. For example, when we approach an authority figure sitting at a desk the distance and speed of approach is determined by status. Those with high status walk directly to the desk, those with low status remain near the door until encouraged to come closer.

Space is a status signal in an office. Desks may be purposefully large to hold visitors at a respectable distance.

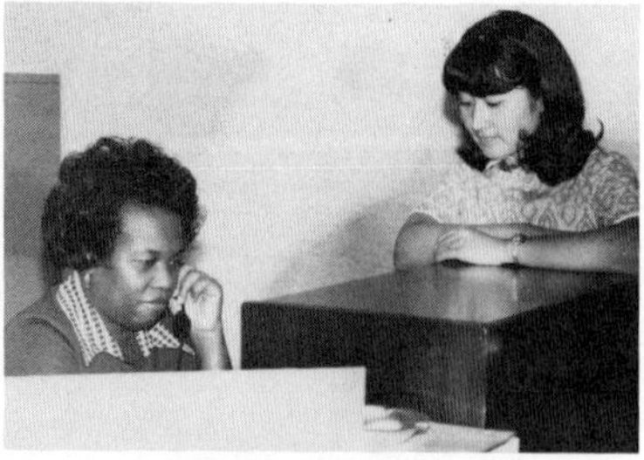

The desk, however, of a person who serves the public is not viewed in the same manner and people freely walk directly to it.

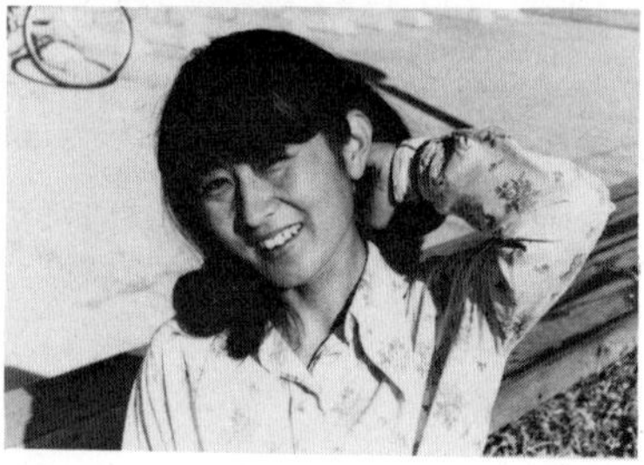

Presentations related to sexuality are interesting to nearly everyone. Men and women have particular body language mannerisms, called grooming *or* preening *gestures that indicate,*

"I am interested. I like you. Notice me; I am an attractive person."

"I am interested in you and I want to relate to you, but this is not a sexual matter."

Grooming mannerisms cannot be done without some risk of rejection and we are taught cultural ways of timing them. We react to the same mannerism differently according to the speed or subtlety with which it is made.

Women groom by pushing the hair away from their face.

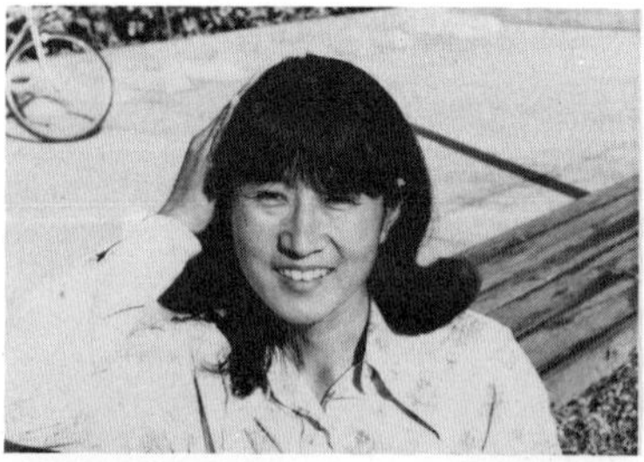

By stroking their hair and by rearranging their clothes and checking their makeup.

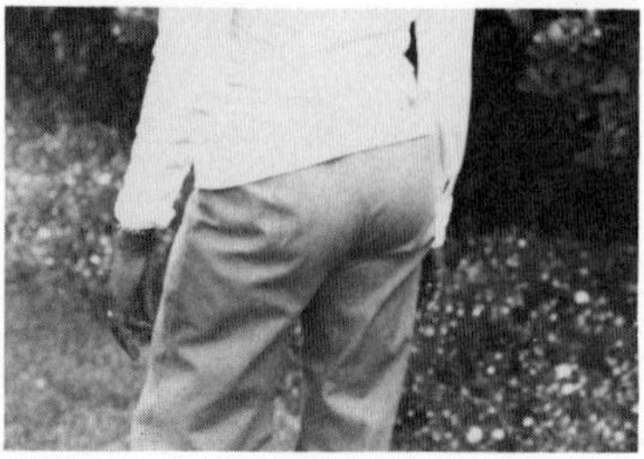

Walking with a hip roll is also a grooming mannerism.

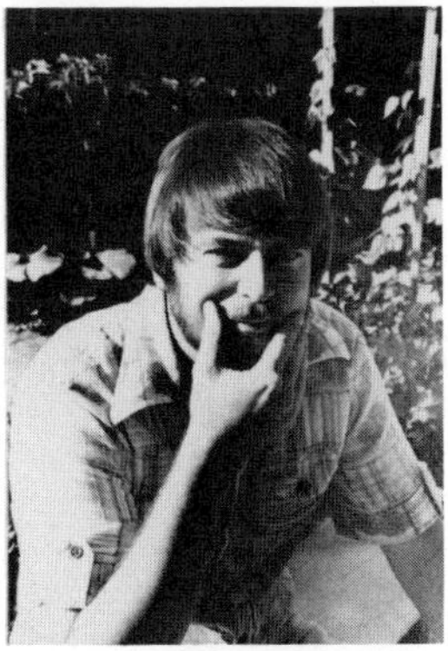

Men groom by stroking a beard or combing their hair.

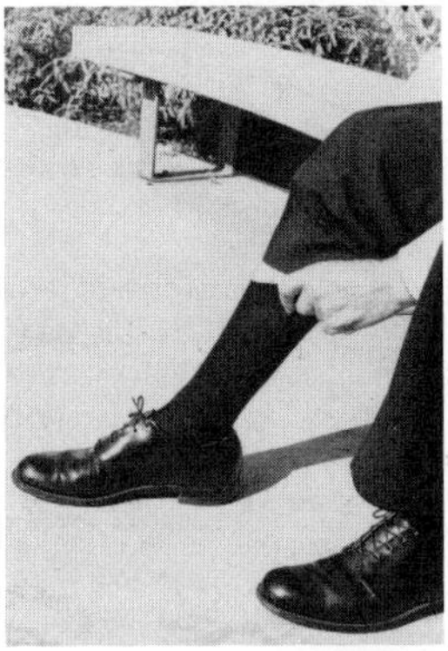

They pull up their socks and arrange their tie.

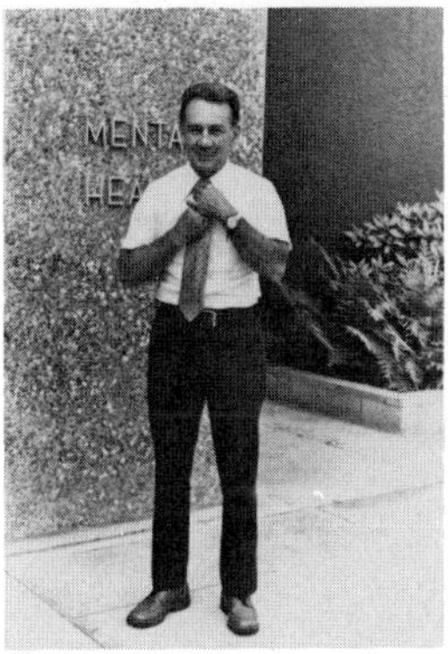

They also typically suck in their stomach, square their shoulders and rearrange their clothing.

Clothing too, sends messages and research shows that clothing does make a difference as to how people respond to others. Clients sometimes feel that wearing a hospital gown puts them in a 1 down position.

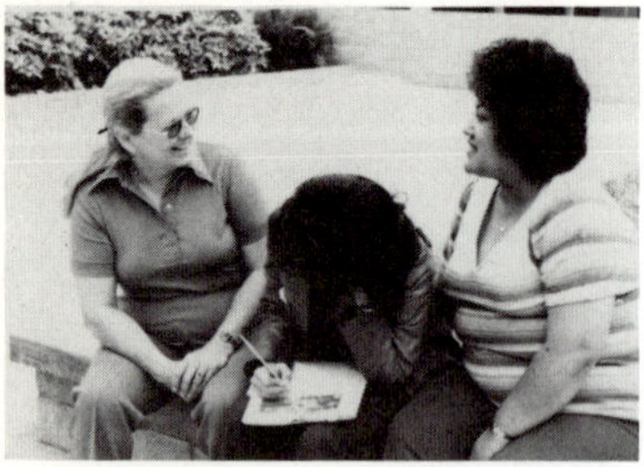

When people are in groups they also rapidly form territorial areas. They space themselves to form circles, squares, or triangles. Sometimes the furniture determines the arrangement.

In this situation the woman in the middle is blocked off as the others strive to form a conversational bond. The setting does not permit a normal triangle to form.

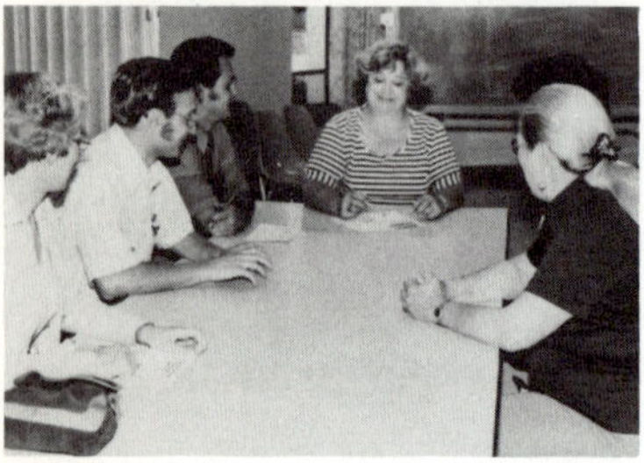

In a small group the dominant member usually sits at the head of the table or becomes the center of focus of a circle.

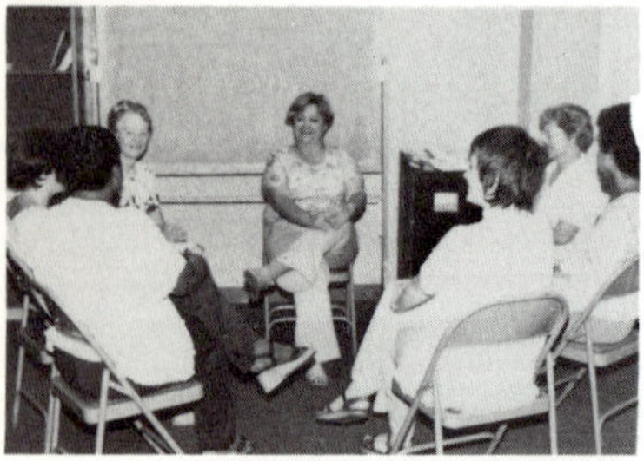

Generally the leader of the group influences the posture and position of other group members. When she crosses her legs, others generally follow suit.

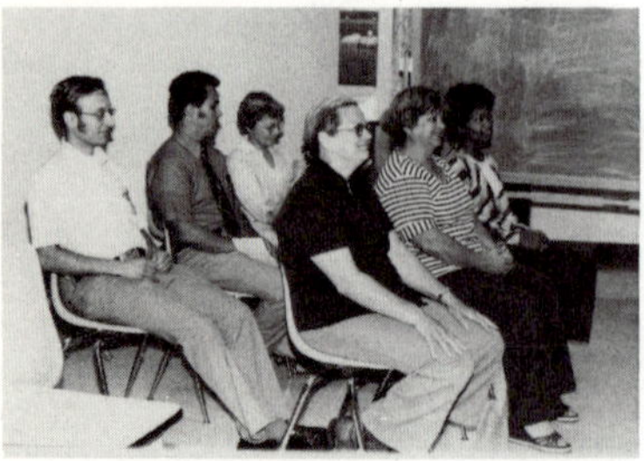

It is interesting to observe students in a classroom for similar and different positions and how and when positions change. Notice how rapidly students determine their own territories.

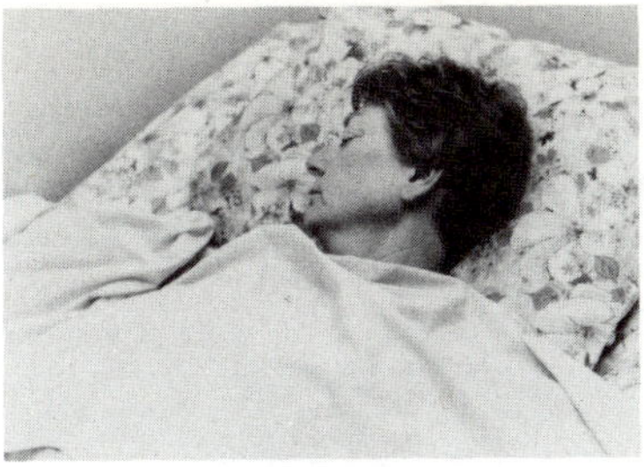

The importance of body language is just as relevant to the client in the hospital as it is to anyone else. For example, this woman may be sleeping or she may be turning away from the staff and expressing anger, isolation, or sadness.

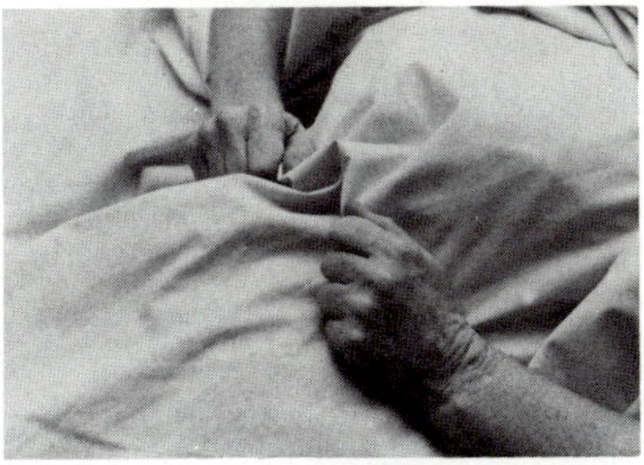

These hands may be clutching the bed linen in pain or anxiety or fear or anger or confusion.

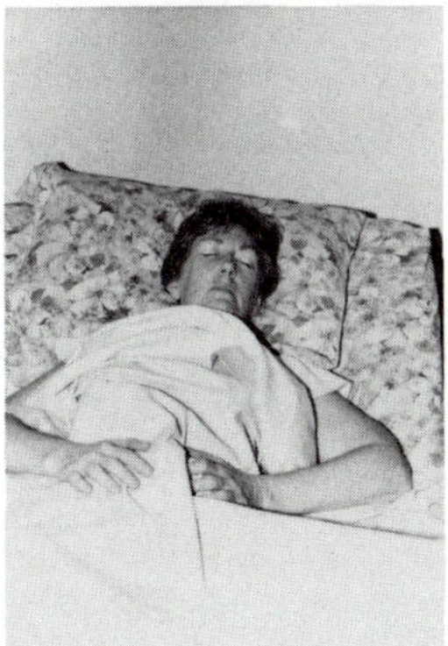

When you enter this room you can immediately observe that this woman is experiencing discomfort in the abdomen.

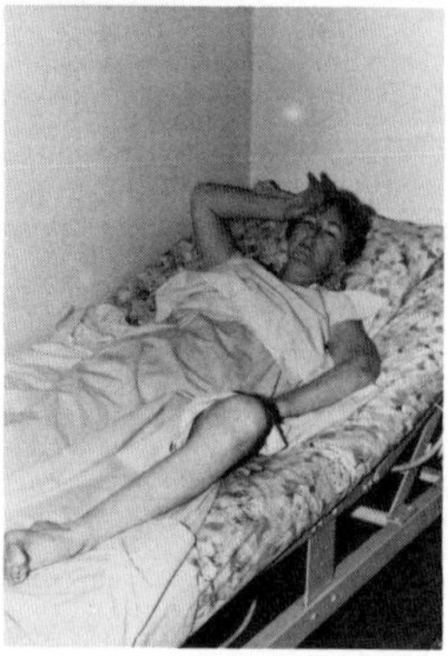

When the client exposes her body it is very important to collect data to determine why. It may simply be that the room is too warm or it may indicate confusion, anxiety or pain.

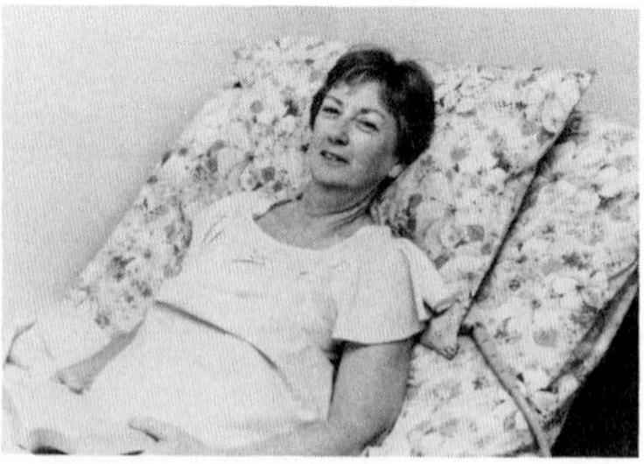

Most of us want to see a smiling client, yet sometimes nurses avoid a client who looks like this because they feel they are not needed. Careful observation of verbal and nonverbal communication will show that these clients have needs too.

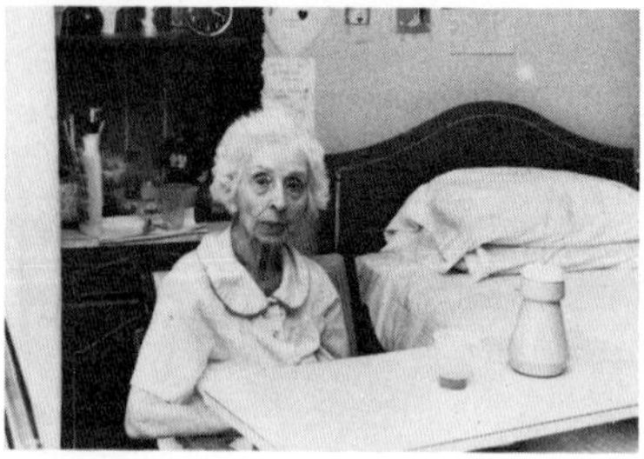

In a hospital the client's territory includes a bed and bedside table. It is important to remember the client will appreciate our consideration of their personal space. It is interesting to observe the way in which this territory quickly reflects messages about the client.

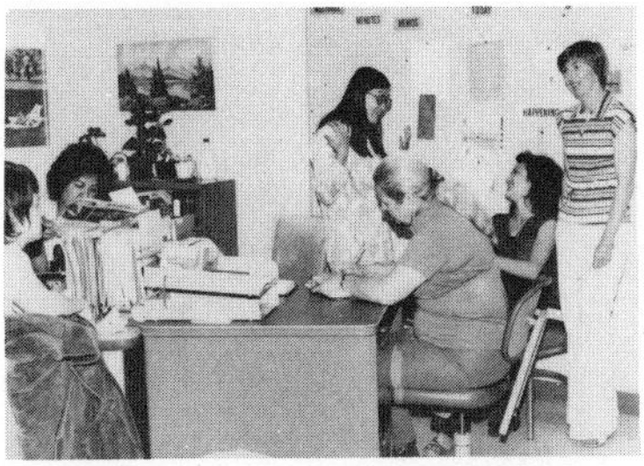

Now you have some clues as to how to read body language a little better when you view the world and the people in it.

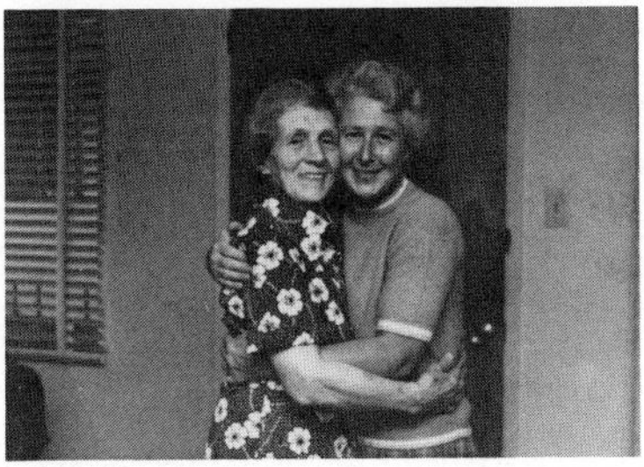

If we were to accurately read every body language message, be aware of all points, postures and presentations, we would be exhausted. It is reasonable, however, to increase our awareness considerably by carefully watching the people we are communicating with in more than a casual way. Experienced nurses view body language and nonverbal communication as essential to complete assessment of a client.

In closing, remember that messages from one person to another are qualified by: (1) the context in which they take place; (2) verbal context; (3) vocal and linguistic patterns; and (4) body movements.

Posttest

1. List three variables that influence body language.

   A.

   B.

   C.

2. The messages from one person to another are qualified by:

   A. the context in which they take place

   B. verbal context

   C. vocal and linguistic patterns

   D. ethnic background

   E. body movements

3. Define "points" in body language.

4. Describe at least three different points and their common meanings.

   A.

   B.

   C.

5. Describe what a change in position may mean during a conversation.

6. Define "presentation" in body language.

7. List at least three variables that determine social distance during a conversation.

   A.

   B.

   C.

8. Describe how status affects the way in which one approaches someone sitting at a desk.

9. List two grooming mannerisms for men and two for women.

Men	*Women*
A.	C.
B.	D.

10. Describe at least four common body language messages sent by clients to nurses.

A.	C.
B.	D.

Posttest Answers

1. A. ethnic background B. social class C. personal style
2. A, B, C, E
3. Points are movements of the head, face, and hands.
4. Any points of the head, face and hands and a reasonable meaning are acceptable.
5. A change in position may mean A. a need for more comfort B. change by habit C. disagreement with the speaker D. a desire to assume a new approach E. a desire to remove oneself from the communication.
6. All of the positions a person goes through in the course of a conversation is called a presentation.
7. A. ethnicity B. level of intimacy C. prior relationship D. the business they have together E. available space F. circumstances
8. Those with high status walk directly to the desk, those with less status wait to be invited to come closer.
9. A. pulling up socks, or arranging tie B. stroking beard, combing hair or rearranging clothing. C. pushing hair away from face or checking makeup D. walking with a hip roll or rearranging clothing
10. anger, withdrawal, isolation, sadness, fear, anxiety, pain, anticipation, confusion

REFERENCES

1. Ardrey, Robert. *The Territorial Imperative* (New York: Atheneum, 1966).
2. Fast, Julius. *Body Language* (New York: Pocket Books, 1970).
3. Hall, Edwart T. *The Silent Language* (Greenwich, Connecticut: Fawcett Publications, 1959).
4. Kron, Thora. *Communication in Nursing* (Philadelphia: W.B. Saunders Company, 1972).
5. Lewis, Garland K. *Nurse-Patient Communication* (Dubuque, Iowa: Wm. C. Brown Company, 1973).
6. O'Brien, Maureen J. *Communications and Relationships in Nursing* (Saint Louis: C.V. Mosby Company, 1974).
7. Scheflin, Albert E., and Alice Scheflin. *Body Language and Social Order* (Englewood Cliffs, New Jersey: Prentice-Hall, Inc., 1972).

Termination

DIRECTIONS

1. Complete the pretest. If you answer all the questions correctly, you may choose to complete the unit on termination for added enrichment and knowledge.
2. After the pretest, complete the activities as directed. The activities and exercises should be completed in the order presented.
3. In order to complete the unit, you will need a pencil or pen. No other materials are needed.
4. A posttest will be given at the end of the unit. Successful completion of this test is necessary for you to have met the unit objectives.

OBJECTIVES

Upon completion of this unit on termination, the learner will be able to:

1. Define termination.
2. List at least ten words, ideas, or synonyms associated with termination.
3. Describe the concept *separation anxiety.*
4. Identify five stresses associated with termination.
5. Identify five possible responses to stresses of termination.
6. Describe three possible outcomes of the termination process.
7. Compose six positive outcomes of termination for both client and nurse.
8. Formulate a nursing intervention for dealing with termination of a nurse-client relationship.

Pretest

True (T) or False (F)

_____ 1. Termination, most commonly, refers to an abrupt finish or conclusion of an event.

_____ 2. Departure, limit, and infinite are supportive of the concept of termination.

_____ 3. Since the client may need the nurse's services in the future, most nurse-client relationships should be inconclusive.

_____ 4. Separation anxiety is related to the loss of any loved object and the pain of mourning.

_____ 5. Theorists generally agree that early developmental experiences have minimal effect on how an individual will handle termination as an adult.

_____ 6. Since it indicates "finding" a loved object, getting married seldom precipitates separation anxiety.

_____ 7. It is *not* imperative for a nurse to know all of a client's early experiences with termination.

_____ 8. Loneliness, helplessness, and conflict are all stresses that might be precipitated by termination.

_____ 9. Sadness and withdrawal are common responses to the stress of termination, but anger is seldom manifested.

_____10. Termination is often avoided by both client and nurse.

_____11. The client is the one who usually has the most difficulty with termination.

_____12. Termination can be a learning experience, and produce growth, for both client and nurse.

_____13. Termination "work" should be initiated at the very beginning of a nurse-client relationship.

_____14. Nurses often make termination more difficult by promoting overdependency of the client.

_____15. It is important that both nurse and client recognize their relationship as a finite working one.

Pretest Answers

1. False 2. False 3. False 4. True 5. False 6. False 7. True
8. True 9. False 10. True 11. False 12. True 13. True 14. True
15. True

INTRODUCTION

What we call the beginning
is often the end and to make an end
is to make a beginning.
The end is where we start from.
T. S. Eliot

A dictionary definition of *termination* would be—the end of something in space or time. Keep this in mind as you read the following quotes and sayings.

The end crowns all;
And that old common arbitrator, time
Will one day end it.
SHAKESPEARE

All's well that ends well,
still the finis is the crown.
SHAKESPEARE

Farewell a word that must be, and hath been,
A sound which makes us linger; -yet- farewell.
BYRON

Abruptness is an eloquence in parting,
When spinning out the time is but the
weaving of new sorrow.
SIR JOHN SUCKLING

We are parted; and every parting
is a form of death, as every
re-union is a type of heaven.
EDWARDS

To die and part
Is a less evil; but to part and live,
There—there's the torment.
LANDSDOWNE

Good night, good night! parting is such sweet sorrow
That I shall say—good night, till it be morrow.
SHAKESPEARE

What came to mind as you read these poetic offerings? In the space provided, list words, ideas, or synonyms that occurred to you and might be readily associated with termination.

1.	6.
2.	7.
3.	8.
4.	9.
5.	10.

Possible responses are below.

This should not have been too difficult. Termination easily suggests:

ending—beginning

parting, departure, farewell

conclusion, completion

limit—final, finish, finite

words from other languages—adieu, adios, arivederci, or more common, goodbye.

SAYING GOODBYE

Each of us has experienced saying goodbye. Give a few moments thought to the most recent goodbye you said to someone or somewhere. Was it unpleasant or pleasant? Leaving a favorite place or special people often brings mixed feelings. There may be excitement about moving to new and different situations; at the same time, sadness may be felt for what is being left behind.

At the risk of stating the obvious, this module deals with the ending of a relationship. More specifically, the relationship in question is that between the nurse and client that develops as a result of their working together. Each time a nurse provides care and services, and a client utilizes them, a working relationship is in effect. As important as beginning such a relationship is ending it in a positive and adaptive manner; thus, termination. Recalling our dictionary definition of termination, the "something ending in space or time" is the finite working relationship between nurse and client.

The ending of any interpersonal relationship can be stressful, bringing about feelings of loss, anxiety or depression. Whenever involvement and closeness develop—as in the nurse-client situation—termination can cause feelings of emotional, or even physical, discomfort. Central to understanding the termination process, and its impact on individuals, is the concept of *separation anxiety.* A brief explanation will be given here. For a more in-depth understanding, you are encouraged to read the *American Journal of* Nursing articles listed in the References (Hale and Richardson, 1963; Travelbee, 1969).

Separation anxiety is the feeling of discomfort, fear, or depression experienced in reaction to the loss of a loved person or object, and includes the pain of mourning such a loss. It is generally agreed that the prototype for this phenomenon is the separation of infant and mother, either at birth or at some point in the early developmental years. The degree of discomfort of early separation experiences, and how they are handled, determine to a great extent how an individual will manage future separations or termination of relationships during his or her entire lifetime. Beginning school commonly precipitates separation anxiety. From what is the child separating? What loss is involved? List other major separation experiences that would likely produce anxiety.

1.

2.

3.

4.

5.

Possible answers are:

1. graduation from school
2. getting a job
3. going to college
4. entering military service

5. getting married
6. divorce
7. illness, hospitalization
8. loss of body part of function
9. death of a loved one
10. death of self

From what we have covered so far, you should be able to recognize that if a nurse is at all successful in working with a client, some separation anxiety is likely at the ending of the relationship. It is important also to recognize that both *client and nurse* will experience anxiety and discomfort since both are involved in the relationship that is concluding. Introspection, self-examination, and self-awareness will aid the nurse in dealing with his or her own feelings, thereby making the nurse more able to help the client cope with his or her stresses.

It is not important for the nurse to know all of a client's experiences of early separations. To understand his or her feelings and behavior though, it is important to realize that the feelings are a revival of feelings of earlier separations and terminations. These feelings may be transferred to the nurse, consciously or unconsciously, and a client may need encouragement to express them. Too, support and reassurance are important to help the client recognize that it is acceptable to express feelings, even negative ones such as anger.

From what we have covered so far, it should be apparent that a variety of stresses may be experienced by the client and/or nurse. Examples of stresses are:

1. fear of – abandonment
   aloneness
   withdrawal of love
   death
2. feeling of – loss
   isolation
   loneliness
   rejection
   helplessness
3. conflict–dependence vs. independence

The responses to these stresses are also varied. Responses may be adaptive or unadaptive, depending mainly on how they are managed. Again, the client *and* nurse will experience feelings and manifest behaviors in response to the stress of separation. The following puzzle will help you to identify a number of responses to termination and separation anxiety. The answers appear before the posttest.

Across

1. a sorrowful state or condition.
2. low spirits, gloominess, dejection.
3. somatic indications of illness or discomfort.
4. the act of retreating or moving back.
5. a strong feeling excited by a real or supposed injury.
6. intense emotional suffering caused by loss or misfortune.
7. the act of shedding tears.

Down

1. the practice or habit of attacking or invading, usually unprovoked.
2. a feeling of enmity, ill will, unfriendliness, or antagonism.

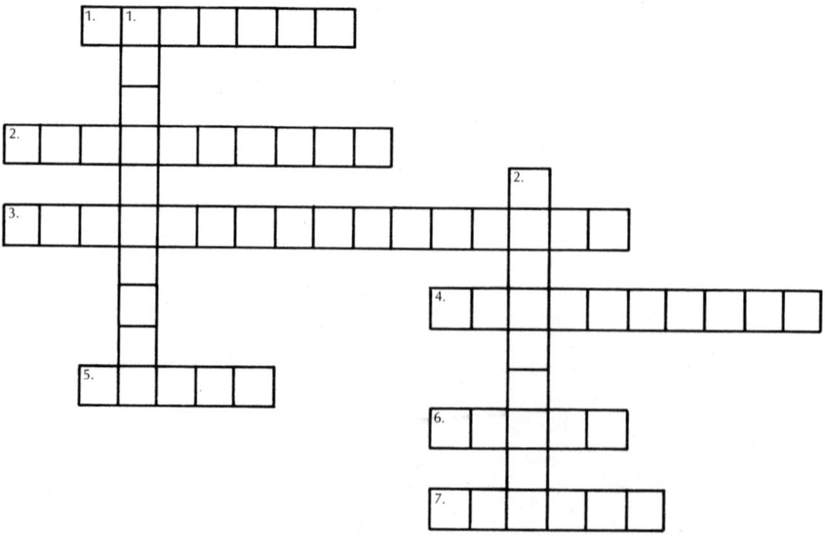

The outcome of the termination process may be that it is essentially aborted; handling the separation may be prolonged or put off, representing problems of the nurse, the client or both. Or mismanaging termination may result in unadaptive behavior by the client or nurse. Basically this would be manifested by the continuing of maladaptive responses to the stress of separation anxiety and termination.

On the other hand, the outcome of termination may well be adaptive. Acceptance of termination, and dealing with concomitant stress, can become a valuable learning experience for the nurse and client resulting in growth and further development.

Based on what you have learned thus far, formulate a *positive* outcome of the termination process for client and nurse in relation to the six processes of living listed below. No answers will be provided, but this exercise will serve as a good review in preparation for the posttest.

Decision Making

Client:

Nurse:

Stress Response

Client:

Nurse:

Learning

Client:

Nurse:

Growth and Development

Client:

Nurse:

Changing

Client:

Nurse:

Communication

Client:

Nurse:

In conclusion, let us review some of the main aspects of the process of termination in nursing practice.

1. Who—client *and* nurse. Who else might be involved in the management of termination?
2. What—the ending of a *finite* working relationship between nurse and client. What might occur if the nurse or client do not acknowledge the limits of their working together?
3. When—ideally, termination "work" should begin at the onset of the nurse-client relationship. When would be the least effective time to begin?
4. Where—a setting providing comfort, privacy, safety, and so on. Where, in the clinical agencies you have been in, can you recall rooms or places appropriate for termination work?
5. Why—so both client and nurse can grow. Why is this important?

6. How—
   a. define relationship explicitly including limits, roles, goals, objectives, and so on.
   b. prepare for termination from the beginning.
   c. nurse should become aware of, and work through, own feelings.
   d. assist the client as needed in dealing with his or her feelings.
   e. be sure to say, Goodbye!

Pearl of Wisdom

One who can successfully say Goodbye,
can say Hello.

You have completed this module. Thank you for your attention and participation. Do the posttest, check your answers, and you will be ready to learn more about the termination process in your clinical practice and interpersonal relationships.

Oh yes—one last word before we part company—Goodbye!

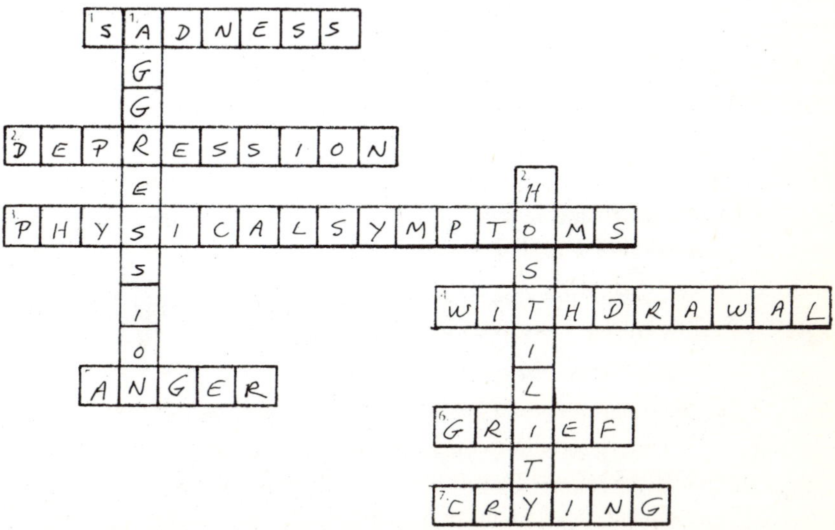

Posttest

Circle the correct answer.

1. Which of the following is the *best* definition of termination?

   A. an abrupt conclusion or finish of an event

   B. the end of something in space or time

   C. the prolonged outcome or result of a situation

   D. the avoidance of limiting or completing a relationship

2. Which of the following are *not* usually associated with termination?

   A. beginning/end

   B. departure

   C. farewell

   D. infinite

   E. limit

   F. inconclusive

   G. adios

   H. unfinished

   I. parting

   J. final

3. The following statements apply to the concept, *separation anxiety.* Are they true (T) or false (F).

   A. Separation anxiety is related to the loss of a loved object and the pain of mourning.

   B. It is generally agreed that separation anxiety *first* occurs when a child is separated from the family by beginning school.

   C. The way in which early separation experiences are handled has little effect on how an individual will manage future separations or termination of friendships during his or her lifetime.

D. Going to college, getting a job, entering military service, and getting married are all events which precipitate separation anxiety.

E. It is important for a nurse to know all about a client's experiences of early separations from significant people.

4. Which of the following are stresses associated with termination?

A. feeling abandoned
B. fear of death
C. loneliness
D. feeling helpless
E. conflict
F. fear of withdrawal of love

1. A only
2. A, C, F
3. all except B and E
4. all except E
5. all of the above

5. Which of the following are common responses to the stress of termination?

A. sadness
B. anger
C. withdrawal
D. aggression
E. somatic symptoms
F. grief

1. A, C, E
2. B, D, E, F
3. all except E
4. all except F
5. all of the above

6. The following statements apply to the outcome or results of termination. Are they true (T) or false (F)?

A. Termination, and concomitant stress, can be easily avoided by both the client and nurse.

B. The nurse's own feelings may affect how the termination is managed.

C. The client most often is the one who has difficulty with termination.

D. If the client is resistive, the nurse can do little to promote an adaptive termination.

E. Accepting, and dealing with, termination can become a learning and growth experience for both client and nurse.

7. Would the following promote a positive outcome of termination for both nurse and client? (Yes or No.)

A. The nurse decided, in order to protect the client from stress, to wait until his or her day of discharge to talk with the client about termination.

B. To deal with his or her own feelings regarding termination, the nurse expressed sadness to the client, for example, "I will miss seeing you when I come to work each day."

C. To learn how to best deal with a client's termination, the nurse sought counsel with the psychiatric nurse consultant.

D. When a client became angry while talking about termination, the nurse told him firmly, "Mr. S., you're acting like a child. Don't take your frustrations out on me. After all, the doctor ordered your discharge."

E. To change a pattern of avoiding talking about termination, a nurse forced him or herself to face the client and stated, "I need to say goodbye."

F. To help a client talk about termination, the nurse pointed out the incongruency between his or her verbal, "I'm glad to be going home," and his or her nonverbal behavior indicating anxiety, withdrawal, and depression.

8. Would the following be considered a positive outcome for a nurse having dealt with termination? (Yes or No.)

A. Deciding to begin dealing with future terminations at the onset of the nurse-client relationship.

B. In the future, keeping all his or her feelings to him or herself so as to better facilitate the client expressing his or hers.

C. Learning that termination should be dealt with in any nurse-client relationship, not only those in a psychiatric setting.

D. Recognizing his or her responsibility to facilitate the client's expressing and dealing with his or her feelings, even the ones difficult to accept, for example, anger.

E. Recognizing the need to change his or her behaviors that were overprotective of the client and promoted the client's dependency on the nurse.

F. Minimizing future conversation with clients, since it promoted closeness and thus made termination more difficult and stressful.

9. Would the following be considered a positive outcome for the client having dealt with a termination? (Yes or No)

A. Deciding to visit the hospital unit once a week for a while to lessen the discomfort of termination.

B. To allow him or herself to cry when he or she felt sad saying goodbye to friends and loved ones.

C. Learning that termination is an inevitable part of living, and it cannot be avoided.

D. Feeling embarrassed for his or her child-like behavior, for example, anger, withdrawal, somaticizing; and firmly resolving to suppress this behavior in the future.

E. Revising his or her mode of relating by terminating future relationships before they become meaningful enough that it would be painful if the other person left.

F. Talking more with his or her teenage son about how much he or she would miss him when he went away to college although he or she realized the son's need to move away from home.

10. The following statements apply to the planning of interventions during the termination process. Are they true (T) or false (F)?

A. It is important that both nurse and client recognize their relationship as a finite working one.

B. It matters very little at what point in the relationship preparation for termination begins.

C. For intensive termination work, a setting providing comfort, privacy, and safety should be available.

D. It is important that the nurse-client relationship remain loose with few limits and roles defined.

E. The nurse should never assume that the client needs to work through termination, but should wait for direct requests for help with this.

F. A final "Goodbye" is an important aspect in termination of the nurse-client relationship.

Posttest Answers

1. B 2. D, F, H 3. A. T B. F C. F D. T E. F 4. 5 5. 5
6. A. T B. T C. F D. F E. T 7. A. No B. Yes C. Yes
D. No E. Yes F. Yes 8. A. Yes B. No C. Yes D. Yes E. Yes
F. No 9. A. No B. Yes C. Yes D. No E. No F. Yes 10. A. T
B. F C. T D. F E. F F. T

REFERENCES

1. Hale, Shirley L., and Julia H. Richardson. "Terminating the Nurse-Patient Relationship," *American Journal of Nursing* (63: Sept., 1963), 116–119.

2. Kalkman, Marion E. *Psychiatric Nursing* 3rd ed. (New York: McGraw-Hill Book Co., 1967), pp. 236–240.

3. Nehren, Jeanette, and Naomi R. Gilliam. "Separation Anxiety," *American Journal of Nursing* (65: Jan., 1965), 109–112.

4. Travelbee, Joyce. "The Nurse-Patient Relationship, Part IV—Termination," *Intervention in Psychiatric Nursing* (Philadelphia: F.A. Davis Co., 1969), pp. 162–176.

Index

Use it now
as a study guide for your clinical nursing courses.

Use it later
when you review for your **R.N. State Board.**

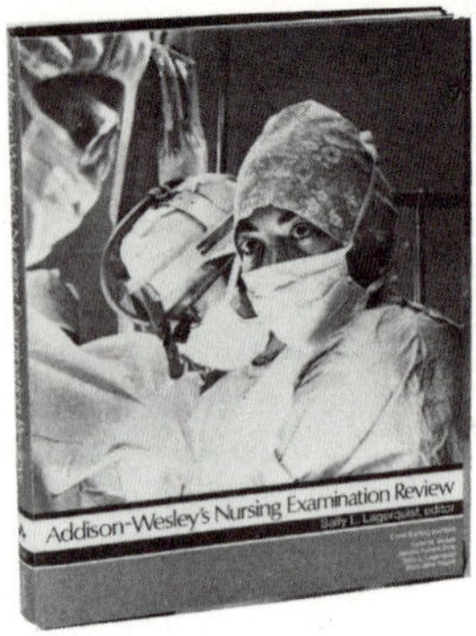

Addison-Wesley's Nursing Examination Review

Sally L. Lagerquist, editor

Contributing authors

Sally L. Lagerquist, R.N., M.S.
University of California, San Francisco

Mary Jane Sauvé, R.N., M.S.
California State College, Sonoma

Irene M. Bobak, R.N., M.N., M.S.N.
San Francisco State Univ., San Francisco

Sandra Forrest Fritz, R.N., M.N.
University of California, Los Angeles

- Covers **Psychiatry, Medicine, Surgery, Pediatrics,** and **Maternity.**
- Presents content in **outline form** for easy identification of what you need to study.
- Contains **numerous situational questions** with answers.
- Includes **Answer Rationales** that fully explain the reasoning behind all answers—a feature most other review books do not have.
- Also includes **annotated Bibliographies,** extensive **Appendices,** and a **special Orientation section** that provides helpful hints for preparing for and taking the State Board.

8½ x 11; 496 pages; hardbound, $12.95
Price subject to change

Order from your local bookstore or order directly from:
Addison-Wesley Medical/Nursing Division, 2727 Sand Hill Road, Menlo Park, CA 94025